GAIL DUFF
HIGH-FIBRE COOKERY

HAMLYN

CONTENTS

We would like to thank:
Frank Hogben & Son, Charing, Kent. Honesty Wholefoods, Union Street, Maidstone, Kent. Brian Cook & Son, Charing, Kent. Lurcocks of Lenham, Lenham, Kent. Valerie Clarke. Nadia Miante. Maggie Wire. Habitat Designs Ltd.

Produced by New Leaf Productions
Photography by Mick Duff
Design by Jim Wire
Series Editor: Sarah Wallace

First published in 1984 by Hamlyn Publishing
Bridge House, London Road,
Twickenham, Middlesex, England

© Copyright Hamlyn Publishing 1984
a division of The Hamlyn Publishing Group Limited

Fifth impression 1986

ISBN 0 600 20809 5
Printed in Spain

Larsa D. L. TF. 930 – 1984

NOTE
1. Metric and imperial measurements have been calculated separately. Use one set of measurements only as they are not exact equivalents.

2. All spoon measures are level unless otherwise stated.

3. Always pre-heat the oven to the given temperature. Cooking times may vary according to the oven. For fan-assisted ovens cooking times may be shorter, so always follow manufacturers' instructions.

4. All recipes serve 4 unless otherwise stated.

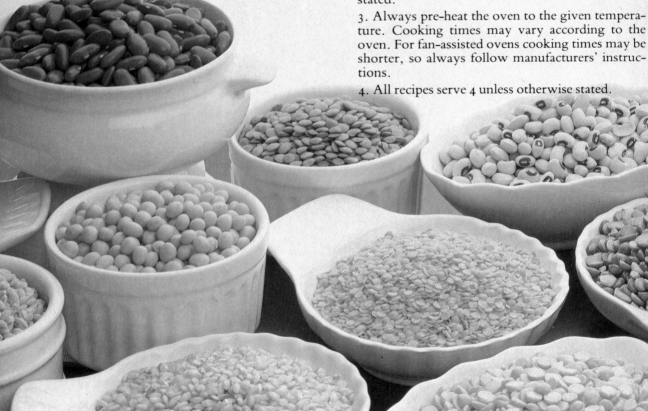

INTRODUCTION

What is fibre?

Fibre is found in all plant foods, be they cereals, fruits or vegetables. It makes up the walls of the plant cells and there are many different types, some strong and rigid and others weak and flexible. When we eat foods containing fibre, the fibre itself is not digested and for many years it was known as 'unavailable carbohydrate' and regarded as unimportant. We now know that fibre or 'roughage', as it is sometimes referred to, has a vital part to play in keeping us healthy.

Why is fibre in the diet important?

As fibre moves through our digestive system it absorbs a great deal of water and as a result all waste matter becomes large, soft and bulky. This means that it can be pushed along the digestive system quickly and easily and food will pass through the body in 12 to 24 hours. Waste matter from a low-fibre diet is small and hard and can take anything up to one week to be eliminated.

Quickly moving waste matter means that any harmful substances that it may contain do not have a chance to be re-absorbed back into the body. Neither can they irritate or inflame the walls of the digestive tract.

A large percentage of fibre in the diet ensures that any bacteria existing in the digestive tract will be beneficial and will work to give us a resistance to certain diseases. A low-fibre diet produces bacteria which are less efficient and which may well increase our liability to certain digestive troubles.

There are many complaints and diseases which have recently been proved to be caused by the slow passage of low-fibre waste. These include constipation, haemorrhoids, diverticular disease, appendicitis and varicose veins.

Sugary, low-fibre foods are also responsible for the fact that dental decay is one of the most common diseases in the Western world, whereas high-fibre foods are thought to contain substances which actually stop the build-up of plaque on the teeth and the subsequent decay.

Research has shown that a high-fibre diet may well reduce cholesterol levels in the body and therefore make related diseases such as gallstones and heart complaints less likely.

Why does fibre help to reduce weight?

In natural plant foods sugars and carbohydrates are bound up with vitamins and minerals and a large percentage of fibre. When these foods are refined, for example by removing the germ and the outer coating of bran from wheat grains to produce white flour, the sugars then make up the main part of the end product.

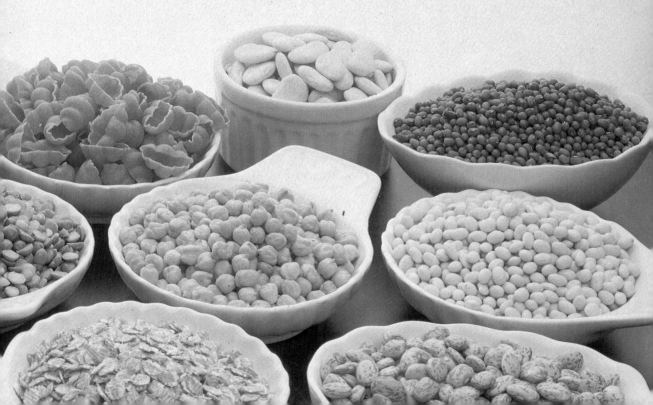

Without the fibre the refined product contains more calories by weight than the original food. The sugars in these refined foods are absorbed very quickly by the body, giving us a quick surge of satisfaction and energy. Unfortunately, without the bulk of the fibre this feeling does not last for very long. We are therefore tempted to eat more and eventually we will take in too many calories for our immediate needs and the excess will be stored as fat.

If high-fibre foods such as wholemeal bread or fresh fruits and vegetables are eaten the combination of fibre with the other nutrients ensures that we are eating less sugars for the bulk of food consumed. We chew fibre-rich foods more thoroughly and the saliva that is then mixed with them bulks out the foods when they reach the stomach. The feeling of satisfaction that this produces lasts for a considerable time and thus prevents overeating.

How can we obtain enough fibre?

In order to keep healthy we need 25–30g/1 oz fibre per day. The best way in which to obtain it is to eat a balanced, natural diet containing a wide variety of whole-grain products, fresh fruit and vegetables and pulses. Avoid refined products such as white flour and sugar and all bought products made from them such as biscuits, pies, packet soups, confectionery and instant desserts.

Eat only wholewheat (also called wholemeal) bread, which is made from flour containing 100% of the wheat grain. Choose wholewheat flour for all home baking and buy whole-grain crispbreads. Wholewheat pasta is just as easy to cook as the white kinds and now comes in many different shapes. Brown rice is also easy to cook. The long grain variety is suitable for all savoury dishes and the short or round grain brown rice can be made into milk puddings. You can also try experimenting with more unusual types of grains.

Choose a whole-grain or bran-enriched breakfast cereal with little or no added sugar: or make up your own muesli with a mixture of rolled oats, wheat, barley and rye.

Include fresh fruits or vegetables in every meal. Eat raw fruits as desserts, as a breakfast-time refresher or as between meals snacks. Cook fruit simply or make it into pies or more elaborate sweet dishes. If possible, eat a salad every day, containing a colourful mixture of all the suitable vegetables that you have available. Always have two vegetables besides the potatoes with your main meal. Cook them only lightly so their crunchy texture is retained.

The pulse vegetables (dried beans and lentils) are all very high in fibre. They can be made into main dishes alone or with meat or fish, mixed into salads or made into soups.

Dried fruits also contain plenty of fibre. They can be eaten by children instead of sweets, soaked and gently cooked to make hot or cold desserts, and used in baking and confectionery.

If you include many different kinds of high-fibre foods in your diet there should be no need to eat any extra by way of bran or bran tablets. Reserve these for when you are away from home and cannot choose what you have to eat. Natural fibre foods are more effective than low-fibre foods with a supplement.

Changing over to a high-fibre diet

If your diet has always been one that is low in fibre, change over gradually to high-fibre foods otherwise you may feel uncomfortable for a few weeks. Start by replacing white bread with wholewheat bread and then by always using 100% wholewheat flour for baking. Then change your breakfast cereal for one that is high in fibre.

Give up sugary foods gradually and at the same time increase your fruit intake.

Cut down slowly on the amount of high-protein foods, such as meat and fish, that you include in any one meal, and replace them with high-fibre foods such as vegetables and pulses.

High-fibre foods are not a medicine, neither are they dull and boring. They can be colourful, interesting and full of flavour and will be enjoyed by the whole family.

If you turn to them gradually, high-fibre eating will easily become a way of life.

Planning high-fibre meals

Every day include as many different types of high-fibre food in your meals as possible and vary the type of meals that you have from day to day. Here are some suggestions.

Breakfast Whole-grain cereal or muesli, fresh fruit; or boiled or poached eggs or other protein food on wholewheat toast.

Lunch Large mixed salad containing small amounts of pulses, nuts or cheese; wholewheat bread or crispbreads.

Dinner Meat or fish dish made with other high-fibre ingredients such as vegetables, pulses or cereal; or vegetable or pulse main dish.

Accompany these with lightly cooked fresh vegetables and jacket potatoes or a brown rice or other whole-grain accompaniment.

Base desserts on fresh fruits, dried fruits and nuts. If between meals snacks are wanted have wholewheat sandwiches or biscuits, fresh fruit or confectionery made from dried fruits.

Your Basic Fibre Chart

Food	Grams of fibre per 25g/1 oz	Food	Grams of fibre per 25g/1 oz	Food	Grams of fibre per 25g/1 oz
Almonds	4.1	Brussels sprouts	1.2	Oranges	0.6
Apples		Cabbage		Parsley	2.5
cooking	0.7	boiled	0.7	Parsnips	1.1
eating	0.6	red, raw	1.0	Peanuts	2.3
Apricots (raw, weighed)		white, raw	0.8	Pears	0.6
dried, raw	6.7	winter, boiled	0.8	Peas	
with stones	0.5	Carrots	0.8	canned	1.8
Artichokes, globe	0.3	Cauliflower	0.6	fresh	1.5
Asparagus	0.4	Celery	0.5	frozen	2.2
Aubergines	0.7	Chicory	0.4	split, dried	3.3
Avocado	0.6	Chinese leaves	0.6	Peppers, green	0.3
Bananas (flesh only)	1.0	Coconut		Pineapple	0.3
Bean sprouts (raw)	0.3	desiccated	6.6	Plums	0.6
Beans		fresh	3.8	Potatoes	0.6
black-eyed, dry weight	7.2	Corn on the cob	1.3	Prunes	3.8
butter, dry weight	6.0	Courgettes	0.5	Raspberries	2.1
chickpeas, dry weight	4.2	Currants	1.8	Redcurrants	2.3
haricot, dry weight	7.2	Dates	2.4	Rhubarb	0.7
mung, dry weight	6.2	Figs	5.2	Rice, brown	1.2
red kidney, dry weight	7.0	Flour, wholewheat	2.7	Spinach	1.8
soya, dry weight	1.2	Gooseberries	0.9	Spring greens	1.1
Beans (fresh)		Grapefruit	0.2	Strawberries	0.6
broad	1.2	Leeks	0.9	Sultanas	2.0
French	0.9	Lentils	3.3	Swedes	0.8
runner	1.0	Mushrooms	0.7	Sweetcorn	1.3
Beetroot	0.7	Oatmeal	2.0	Tomatoes	0.4
Blackberries	2.0	Onions		Turnips	0.8
Blackcurrants	2.4	large	0.4	Walnuts	1.5
Bread, wholewheat	2.4	spring	0.9	Wheatgerm	0.6

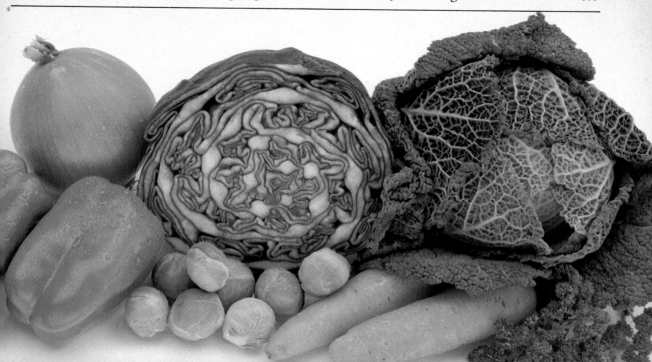

BREAKFASTS

Start the day right with a high-fibre breakfast. There are many bran cereals available for you to choose from and also different varieties of muesli mixtures. If you find these too sweet, buy a muesli base and add fruits and nuts to taste. You can also buy the ingredients to make up the base and mix your own. This base is extremely versatile. Not only can you mix it into a conventional muesli, you can also make it into a crunchy cereal and nut mixture which stores well and which costs much less than the bought kinds.

If you like a hot cereal breakfast, make porridge from coarsely ground oatmeal. Save cooking time in the morning by soaking the oatmeal overnight.

Toast is always a breakfast-time favourite. Make sure that it is always made from wholewheat bread. Serve it plainly with honey or sugar-free marmalade, or make it the base for a savoury breakfast.

Pancakes are quick and easy to cook and these, too, can be served in both sweet and savoury ways. Make the batter the night before to save time. Always use wholewheat flour and for a change mix it with an equal proportion of either cornmeal or buckwheat flour, both of which you can buy in wholefood shops.

MUESLI BASE

450g/1 lb jumbo rolled oats
350g/12 oz rolled wheat
350g/12 oz rolled barley
350g/12 oz rolled rye

Thoroughly mix the rolled cereals together. Store in an airtight container.

CINNAMON FRUIT MUESLI

75g/3 oz dried apricots
75g/3 oz prunes
300ml/½ pint natural apple juice
100g/4 oz muesli base
600ml/1 pint natural yoghurt
½ tsp ground cinnamon
2 oranges
2 dessert apples
1 banana

Put the apricots and prunes into a bowl with the apple juice. Mix the muesli base with the yoghurt and cinnamon. Leave overnight.

In the morning, peel and chop the oranges, chop the apples and slice the banana. Drain the dried fruit. Mix the fresh and dried fruits into the muesli base adding the remaining apple juice to taste to make a fairly moist mix.

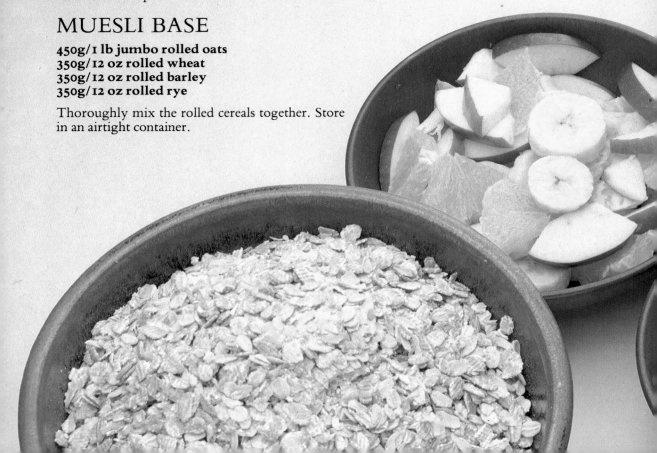

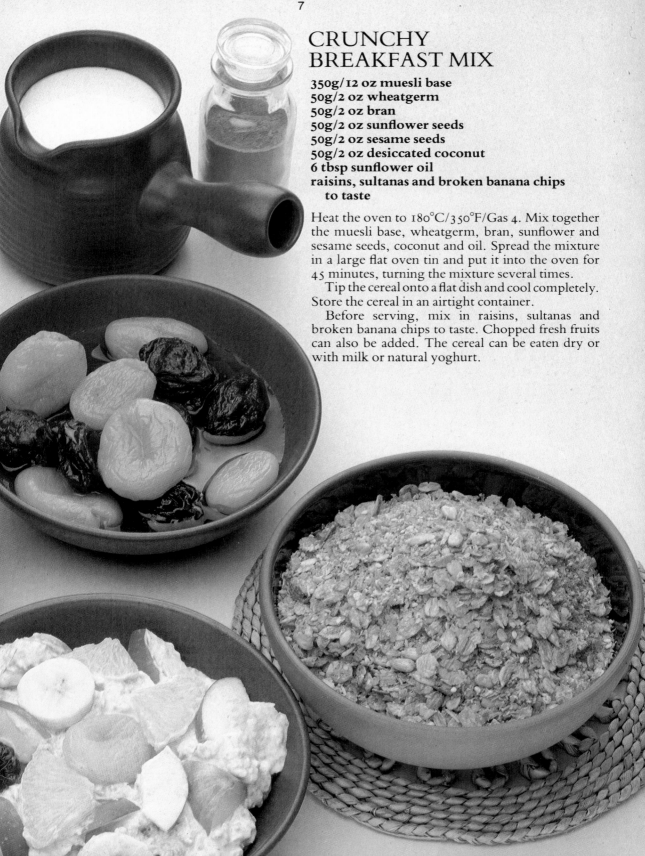

CRUNCHY BREAKFAST MIX

350g/12 oz muesli base
50g/2 oz wheatgerm
50g/2 oz bran
50g/2 oz sunflower seeds
50g/2 oz sesame seeds
50g/2 oz desiccated coconut
6 tbsp sunflower oil
raisins, sultanas and broken banana chips
    to taste

Heat the oven to 180°C/350°F/Gas 4. Mix together the muesli base, wheatgerm, bran, sunflower and sesame seeds, coconut and oil. Spread the mixture in a large flat oven tin and put it into the oven for 45 minutes, turning the mixture several times.

Tip the cereal onto a flat dish and cool completely. Store the cereal in an airtight container.

Before serving, mix in raisins, sultanas and broken banana chips to taste. Chopped fresh fruits can also be added. The cereal can be eaten dry or with milk or natural yoghurt.

APPLE AND BANANA CRUNCH

450g/1 lb cooking apples
50g/2 oz honey
pinch ground cloves
3 tbsp water
2 bananas
100g/4 oz crunchy breakfast mix or a similar
   bought cereal
150ml/¼ pint natural yoghurt

Core and chop the apples. Put the apples into a saucepan with the cloves, honey and water. Cover and set on a low heat for 15 minutes or until the apples are soft. Leave them to cool overnight.

Next morning, heat the oven to 200°C/400°F/Gas 6. Divide the apples between 4 small heatproof bowls. Slice the bananas and put them on top. Cover with the breakfast mix. Put the bowls into the oven for 10 minutes.

Serve topped with yoghurt.

OATMEAL PORRIDGE

150g/5 oz coarse oatmeal
1.2 litres/2 pints boiling water
½ tsp salt

Put the oatmeal into a saucepan. Pour the boiling water over the oatmeal and leave to soak overnight.

Next morning bring to the boil, add the salt and boil gently, stirring frequently for 10 minutes or until all the water is absorbed and the porridge is thick.

Serve with natural yoghurt, milk, honey, Barbados sugar or soaked dried fruits.

★ *50g/2 oz sultanas or raisins may be added while the porridge is simmering.*

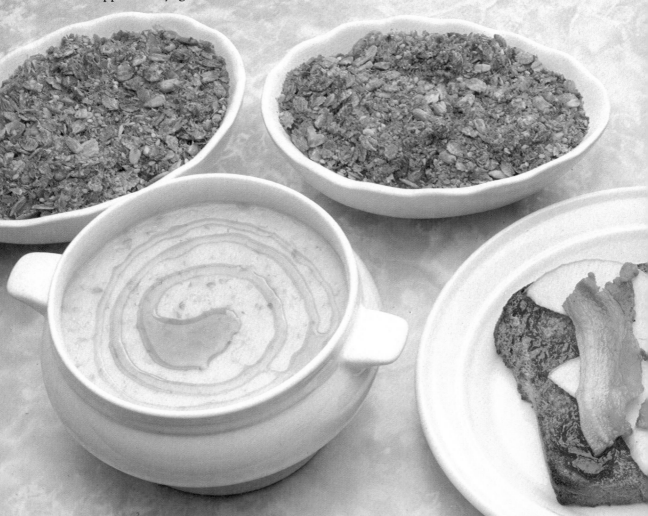

BACON AND APPLES ON TOAST

4 rashers streaky bacon
1 cooking apple
4 slices wholewheat bread
butter
2 tbsp chutney

Cut the rind from the bacon. Cut each rasher in half crossways. Quarter and core the apple and cut into 16 lengthways slices.

Toast the slices of bread on one side only. Turn the slices over, lightly butter and spread with chutney. Lay 4 apple slices on each slice of toast. Put the toast back under the grill for 2 minutes so the apples begin to soften.

Grill the pieces of bacon and put them on top of the apples.

CORN PANCAKES

50g/2 oz cornmeal
50g/2 oz wholewheat flour
¼ tsp sea salt
1 egg
1 egg yolk
1 tbsp oil
150ml/¼ pint milk
150ml/¼ pint water
oil for frying

Put the cornmeal, flour and salt into a bowl. Make a well in the centre. Put in the egg, egg yolk and oil. Beat in a little of the cornmeal and flour from the sides of the bowl. Gradually beat in the milk and water. Leave the batter overnight.

In the morning, make 8 pancakes by frying the batter, 4 tbsp at a time, in hot oil.

Serve either with grilled bacon or scrambled eggs, or with honey or maple syrup.

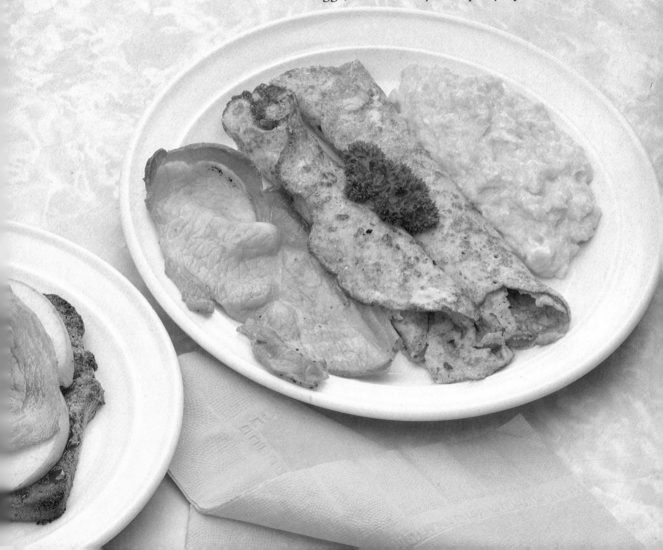

SARDINE AND CHEESE TOASTS

two 120-g/4¼-oz tins sardines in oil
2 tsp tomato purée
pinch cayenne pepper
4 small tomatoes
4 slices wholewheat bread
butter
100g/4 oz smoked Cheddar cheese, grated

Drain and mash the sardines. Mix in the tomato purée and cayenne pepper. Thinly slice the tomatoes. Toast the slices of bread on one side only. Turn over, lightly butter and spread with the sardine mixture. Return to the grill for 2 minutes for the sardines to heat through.

Lay the tomato slices and then the cheese on top. Return to the grill for 1 minute to melt the cheese.

KIPPER CAKES

175g/6 oz kipper fillets
450g/1 lb potatoes
1 medium onion, thinly sliced
4 tbsp milk
3 tbsp chopped parsley
pinch cayenne pepper
25g/1 oz bran
4 tbsp oil

Put the kipper fillets into a bowl. Pour boiling water over the fillets and leave for 15 minutes. Drain. Skin, bone and flake the fish. Scrub the potatoes. Boil the potatoes in their skins, with the onion, until tender. Drain. Skin and mash the potatoes with the onion.

Mix the kippers with the potatoes and beat in the milk, parsley and cayenne pepper. Form the mixture into 8 round flat cakes. Coat in the bran and brush with oil.

Heat the grill to high. Lay the cakes on the hot rack and grill for 3 minutes on each side.

★ *These cakes can be made the night before and brushed with oil just before cooking.*

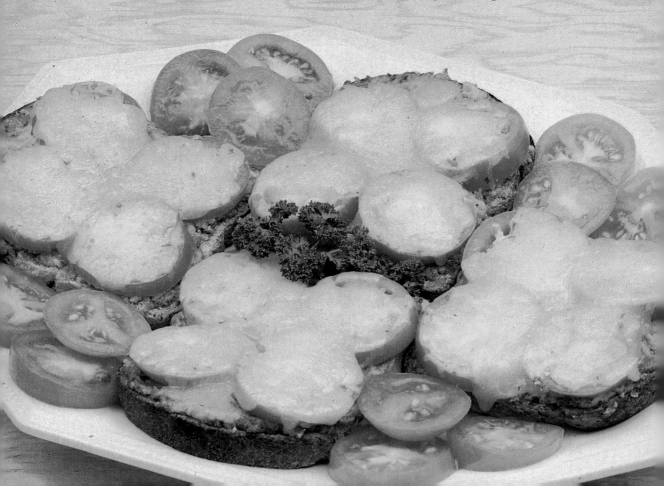

BACON AND PRUNE KEBABS

16 prunes
300ml/½ pint hot strong black tea
8 streaky bacon rashers
wholewheat toast

Soak the prunes in the tea overnight. Next morning, drain and stone them. Cut the rind from the rashers. Cut each rasher in half crossways.

Wrap each prune in a piece of bacon. Thread onto 8 cocktail sticks. Heat the grill to high. Grill the kebabs until the bacon is cooked through, turning several times.

Serve with wholewheat toast.

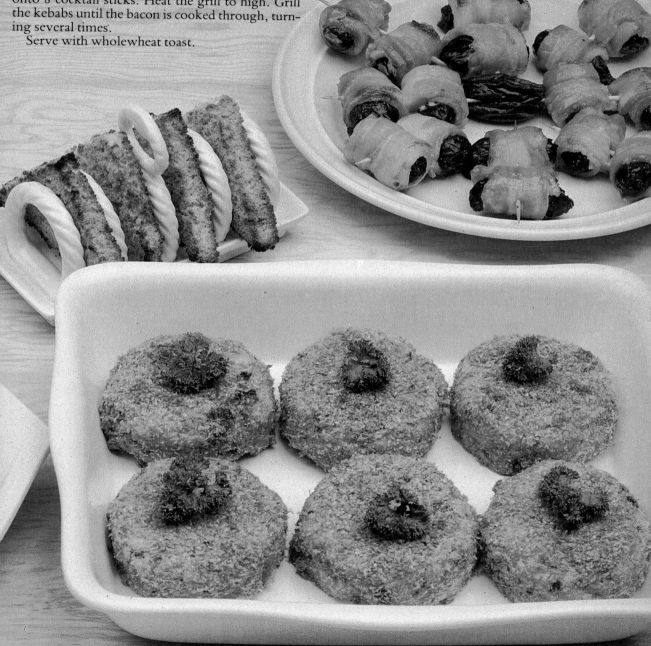

SOUPS AND FIRST COURSES

Soups that contain plenty of fresh vegetables or pulses will naturally be high in fibre. To keep soups healthy, rely mainly on the vegetables themselves for thickening and retain every part of them by either blending or using the blade of the vegetable mill that has the largest holes.

Base hot first courses on small amounts of unusual vegetables; attractive appetizing salads can be made from a variety of vegetables, fruits, nuts, pulses and grains.

HEARTY CARROT AND POTATO SOUP

450g/1 lb carrots
225g/8 oz potatoes
1 large onion, finely chopped
25g/1 oz butter
900ml/1½ pints stock
bouquet garni
sea salt
freshly ground black pepper
2 tbsp Worcestershire sauce
1 tbsp tomato purée
2 tbsp chopped parsley

Finely chop the carrots. Peel and finely chop the potatoes. Melt the butter in a saucepan on a low heat. Stir in the carrots, potatoes and onion. Cover and let them sweat for 10 minutes. Pour in the stock and bring to the boil. Add the bouquet garni and season well. Cover and simmer for 20 minutes.

Remove the bouquet garni. Put half the soup into a blender with the Worcestershire sauce and tomato purée and work until smooth. Stir into the rest of the soup and add the chopped parsley. Reheat, if necessary, before serving.

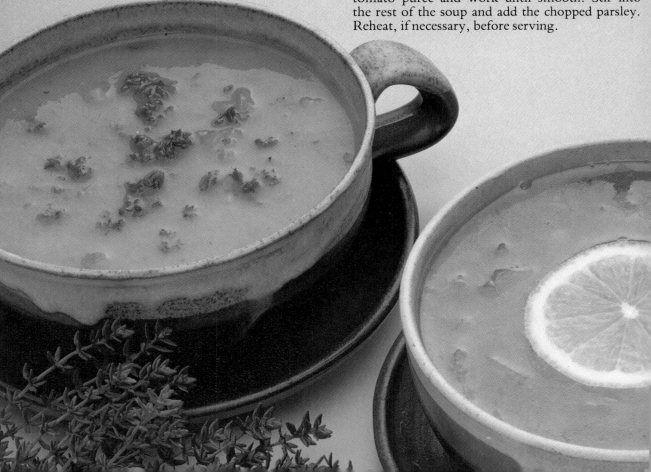

SPICED LENTIL SOUP

4 tbsp oil
1 large onion, thinly sliced
1 garlic clove, finely chopped
2 tsp cumin seeds
1 tsp ground coriander
¼ tsp cayenne pepper
100g/4 oz split red lentils
4 cloves
1.2 litres/2 pints stock
1 bayleaf
4 slices of lemon

Heat the oil in a saucepan on a low heat. Add the onion and garlic and cook until they are soft. Stir in the cumin, coriander and cayenne pepper and cook until the onion begins to brown.

Stir in the lentils and cloves and cook for 1 minute, stirring. Pour in the stock and bring to the boil. Add the bayleaf. Cover and simmer for 45 minutes or until the lentils are soft.

Pour the soup into 4 individual bowls and float a slice of lemon on each one.

BRUSSELS SPROUT AND BACON SOUP

450g/1 lb Brussels sprouts
4 rashers of unsmoked streaky bacon
1 small onion, finely chopped
900ml/1½ pints stock
freshly ground black pepper
2 tbsp chopped savory

Trim and thinly slice the sprouts. Dice the bacon, put into a saucepan and set on a low heat. When the fat begins to run, stir in the sprouts and onion. Cover tightly and let them sweat for 5 minutes. Pour in the stock and bring to the boil. Season with the pepper, cover and simmer for 2 minutes.

Pass the soup through the largest blade of a vegetable mill. Return it to the saucepan, stir in the savory and reheat.

★ *Parsley may be used instead of savory.*

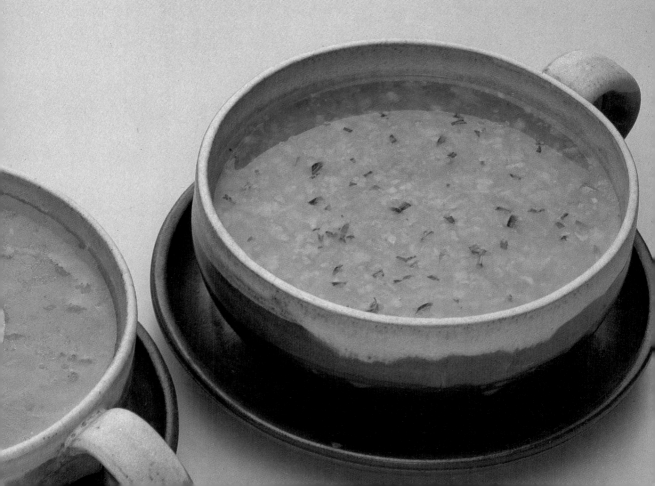

CAULIFLOWER AND APPLE SOUP

1 large cauliflower
1 large cooking apple
900ml/1½ pints chicken stock
1 large onion, thinly sliced
1 tsp curry powder
bouquet garni
150ml/¼ pint natural yoghurt
50g/2 oz shelled walnuts, finely chopped

Break the cauliflower into small florets. Peel, core and slice the apple. Bring the stock to the boil in a saucepan. Put in the cauliflower, apple, onion, curry powder and bouquet garni. Cover and simmer for 20 minutes.

Remove the bouquet garni. Work the soup until smooth in a blender or food processor. Work in the yoghurt. Return the soup to the saucepan and reheat gently, without boiling. Serve in individual bowls with the walnuts scattered over the top.

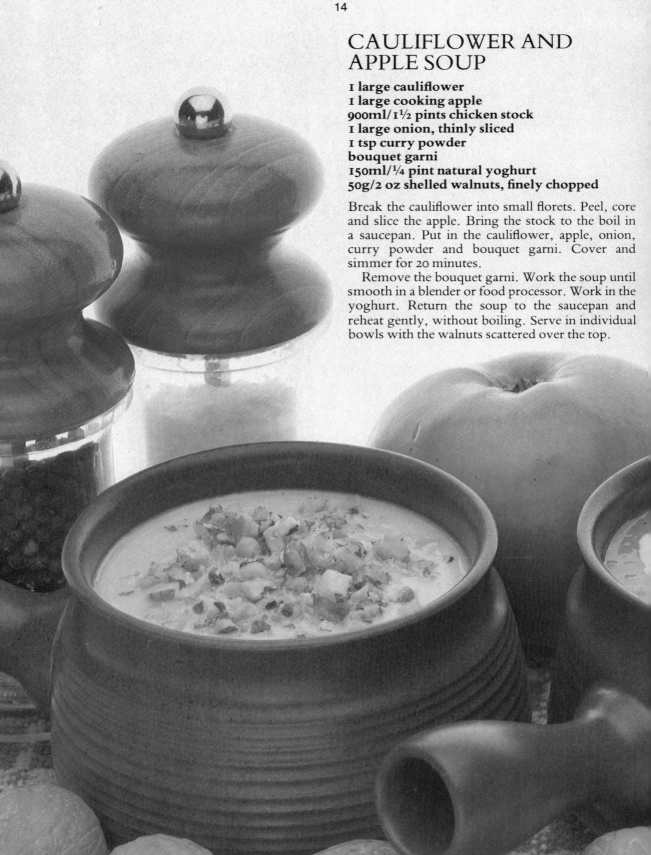

PUMPKIN AND POTATO SOUP

one 900-g/2-lb slice pumpkin
400g/14 oz potatoes
600ml/1 pint ham stock
1 large onion, thinly sliced
bouquet garni
freshly ground black pepper
6 tbsp natural yoghurt

Cut the rind and seeds from the pumpkin. Cut the flesh into 2.5cm/1in chunks. Peel the potatoes and cut into pieces the same size.

Bring the stock to the boil in a large saucepan. Put in the pumpkin, potatoes and onion. Add the bouquet garni and season with pepper. Cover and cook gently for 20 minutes. Remove the bouquet garni.

Work the soup in a blender or food processor until smooth. Reheat if necessary. Serve in small bowls with the yoghurt spooned over the top.

LEEK AND CELERY SOUP

225g/8 oz leeks
4 large celery sticks
25g/1 oz butter
1 tsp wholewheat flour
2 tsp spiced granular mustard
750ml/1¼ pints stock
150ml/¼ pint dry white wine
2 tbsp chopped parsley

Finely chop the leeks and celery. Melt the butter in a saucepan on a low heat. Stir in the leeks and celery. Cover and let them sweat for 7 minutes. Stir in the flour, mustard and stock in that order. Bring to the boil, stirring.

Simmer, uncovered, for 15 minutes. Add the wine and parsley and reheat, without boiling.

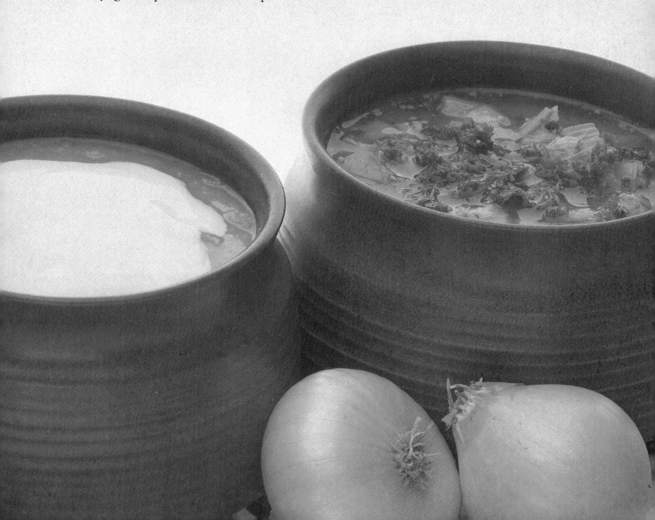

CHILLED PEA AND CHEESE SOUP

900g/2 lb peas (unshelled weight)
40g/1½ oz butter
1 medium onion, finely chopped
900ml/1½ pints chicken stock
sea salt
freshly ground black pepper
100g/4 oz curd cheese
juice of ½ lemon
4 tbsp soured cream
2 tbsp chopped mint

Shell the peas and reserve 10 of the best pods. Melt the butter in a saucepan on a low heat. Stir in the peas and onion, cover and cook for 10 minutes. Pour in the stock and bring to the boil. Season and add the pea pods. Cover the pan and simmer for 15 minutes. Remove the pods.

Put the stock, peas and onion into a blender with the lemon juice and work until you have a pale green liquid. Add the cheese and blend again. Cool the soup then lightly chill it. Pour it into individual bowls and top each one with a portion of soured cream and a little chopped mint.

★ 450g/1 lb frozen peas may be used instead of fresh. To serve hot, reheat the soup gently, without boiling, after adding the cheese.

TABOULEH

175g/6 oz burghul wheat (p.48)
1 small onion, finely chopped
40g/1½ oz parsley, finely chopped
16 black olives, stoned, 8 quartered, 8 halved
4 tbsp olive oil
juice of 1 lemon
sea salt
freshly ground black pepper
8 small tomatoes

Soak the wheat in warm water for 20 minutes. Drain and squeeze dry. Add the onion, parsley and quartered olives. Beat together the oil and lemon juice and season to taste. Mix into the wheat.

Put the wheat in the centre of a flat serving dish and arrange the halved olives on top. Quarter the tomatoes and place around the edge.

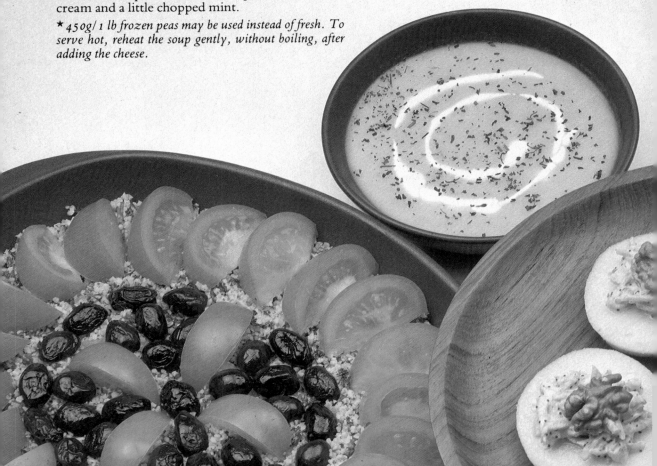

PRAWN AND PEAR SALAD

4 firm Conference pears
juice of 1 lemon
4 tbsp mayonnaise
1 tbsp tarragon mustard
175g/6 oz shelled prawns
8 parsley sprigs

Peel the pears. Brush each one with lemon juice. Cut in half lengthways. Scoop out and discard the cores. Using a teaspoon, scoop out the pears to leave shells about 3mm/⅛in thick. Brush the insides with lemon juice. Chop the scooped out pieces of pear.

   Mix together the mayonnaise and mustard. Add the prawns and pile the mixture into the pears. Garnish each pear-half with a parsley sprig.

APPLE, CARROT AND WALNUT SALAD

4 small Bramley apples
100g/4 oz carrots
50g/2 oz shelled walnuts, chopped
1 tbsp black poppy seeds
6 tbsp natural yoghurt
1 garlic clove, crushed with a pinch of sea salt
freshly ground black pepper
16 walnut halves

Peel and core the apples and cut each one into 4 crossways slices. Arrange the slices, not over-lapping, on 4 small plates.

   Grate the carrots and mix with the chopped walnuts and poppy seeds. Mix the yoghurt with the garlic and pepper and mix into the carrots. Spoon a portion of the carrot mixture onto each apple ring and top with a walnut half.

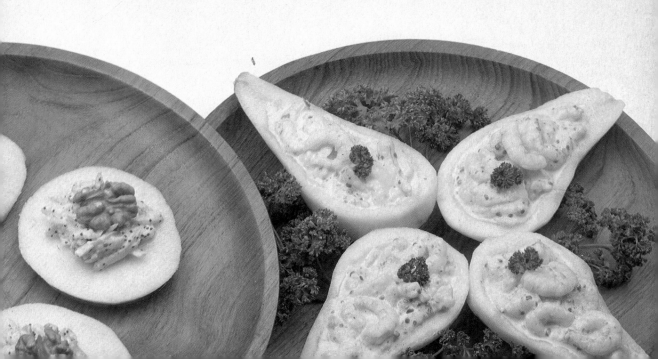

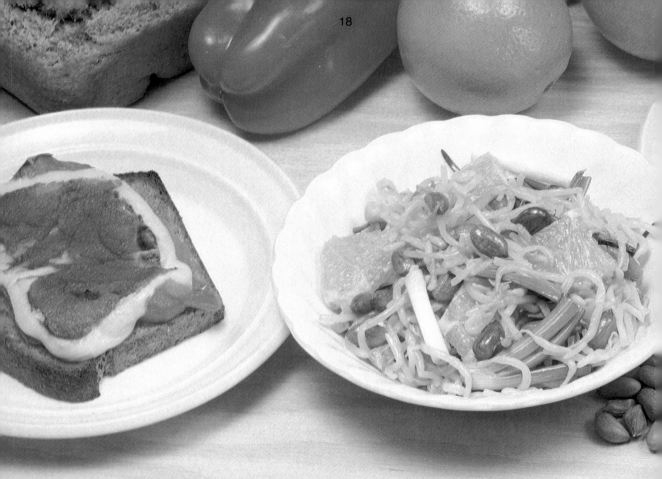

DEVILLED RED PEPPERS

2 large red peppers
2 tbsp tomato purée
2 tsp paprika
¼ tsp Tabasco sauce
175–225g/6–8 oz Edam cheese
4 slices wholewheat bread
butter

Heat the grill to high. Put the peppers under the grill as close to the heat as possible. Char all over and skin the peppers. Cut in half lengthways and remove the cores and seeds. Mix together the tomato purée, paprika and Tabasco sauce.

Toast the bread on one side and butter it on the other. Put the bread back on the grill rack, with a pepper half, cut-side up, on each slice. Cut slices of Edam cheese about 6mm/¼in thick, enough to cover the pieces of pepper. Put slices on top of the pepper halves and spread with the tomato purée mixture. Put the toast under the grill for the cheese to melt (about 2 minutes).

★*Mozarella or Gruyère cheese may be used instead of Edam.*

STIR-FRIED BEAN SPROUTS WITH ORANGES AND PEANUTS

275g/10 oz bean sprouts
12 small spring onions
2 large oranges
3 tbsp oil
garlic clove, finely chopped
50g/2 oz peanuts

Wash and pick over the bean sprouts. Cut the onions into 2.5cm/1in lengths. Peel the oranges and cut into lengthways quarters. Thinly slice. Heat the oil, garlic and peanuts together in a frying pan on a high heat. Stir until the garlic is brown and sizzling.

Put in the bean sprouts and onions and stir for about 1½ minutes until the bean sprouts are just wilted and a good bright green. Mix in the pieces of orange and heat through. Divide everything between 4 individual bowls and serve as soon as possible.

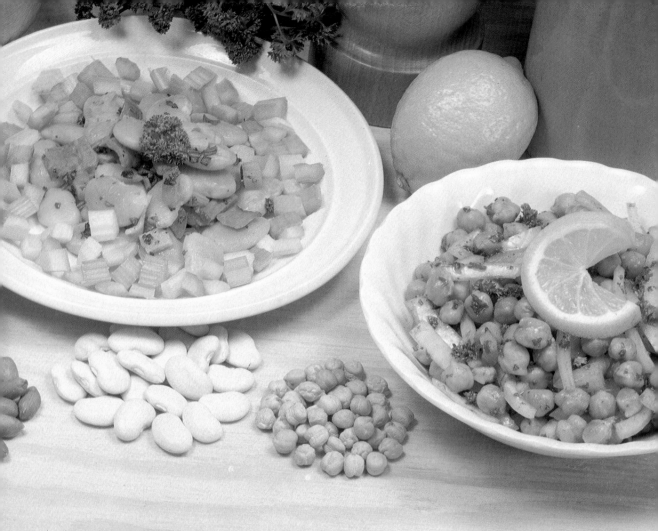

BUTTER BEAN AND BACON SALAD

100g/4 oz butter beans, soaked and cooked
(p.38)
50g/2 oz lean bacon
6 sage leaves, chopped
1 tbsp chopped parsley
4 pickled onions, very finely chopped
2 tbsp oil
1 tbsp cider vinegar
4 celery sticks, chopped
4 parsley sprigs

Put the butter beans into a bowl. Grill the bacon until crisp and chop finely. Mix the bacon into the beans with the herbs and pickled onions. Beat the oil and vinegar together and fold into the beans.

Divide the salad between 4 small plates. Surround each portion with chopped celery and top with a parsley sprig.

CHICKPEA AND ONION SALAD

75g/3 oz chickpeas, soaked and cooked (p.38)
1 medium onion, halved and very thinly sliced
2 tbsp fresh, chopped coriander or parsley
2 tbsp oil
1 tbsp white wine vinegar
2 tsp paprika
¼ tsp cayenne pepper
1 garlic clove, crushed with a pinch of sea salt
4 thin lemon slices

Put the chickpeas into a bowl with the onion and coriander or parsley. Beat the oil, vinegar, paprika, cayenne pepper and garlic together and fold into the chickpeas.

Divide the salad between 4 small bowls and garnish each with a twist of lemon.

FISH

Fish by itself contains no fibre, but it can be mixed with fibre-rich foods to make appetizing meals. Cook fish with vegetables and pulses, make it into pasta dishes, mix it with rice and other grains, or add it to colourful mixed salads.

FISH LASAGNE

575g/1¼ lb white fish fillets
juice of ½ lemon
sea salt
freshly ground black pepper
275g/10 oz wholewheat lasagne
25g/1 oz butter
1 large onion, thinly sliced
3 tbsp wholewheat flour
1 tbsp tomato purée
450ml/¾ pint milk
pinch cayenne pepper
100g/4 oz grated cheddar cheese
450g/1 lb tomatoes, thinly sliced

Heat the oven to 200°C/400°F/Gas 6. Put the fish fillets into a lightly greased dish and sprinkle with lemon juice and seasonings. Cover with foil and bake in the oven for 20 minutes. Skin, bone and flake the fish.

Boil the lasagne in lightly salted water for about 15 minutes until tender. Drain, run cold water through the lasagne and drain again.

Melt the butter in a saucepan on a low heat. Stir in the onion and cook until soft. Stir in the flour, tomato purée and milk.

Bring the sauce to the boil, stirring. Add the cayenne pepper and simmer for 2 minutes. Take the pan from the heat and beat in three-quarters of the cheese.

Put one-third of the lasagne in a layer at the bottom of a 5-cm/2-in deep ovenproof dish. Cover with one-third of the fish, one-third of the tomatoes and one-third of the sauce. Repeat these layers twice more and top with the remaining cheese.

Cook in the oven for 20 minutes or until the top is brown and bubbling.

COD BAKED WITH AUBERGINES

675g/1½ lb cod fillet
2 aubergines, each weighing about 225g/8 oz
6 tbsp olive oil
4 tbsp natural yoghurt
1 tsp ground cinnamon
1 tsp ground paprika
¼ tsp cayenne pepper
1 garlic clove, crushed with a pinch of sea salt
225g/8 oz tomatoes

Heat the oven to 200°C/400°F/Gas 6. Skin the cod and cut into 4 even-sized pieces. Place in the centre of a large serving dish. Cut the aubergines into 1-cm/½-in thick slices. Beat together the oil, yoghurt, spices and garlic.

Brush a little of this mixture over the aubergine slices and arrange the slices round the cod. Spoon the remaining mixture over the cod. Scald, skin and chop the tomatoes and scatter over the top.

Bake the cod for 25 minutes and serve straight from the dish.

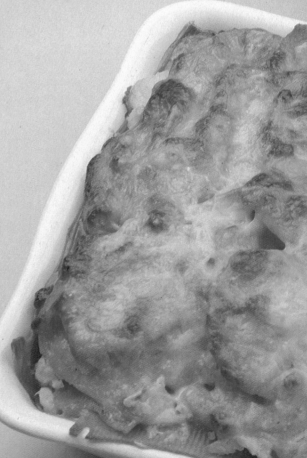

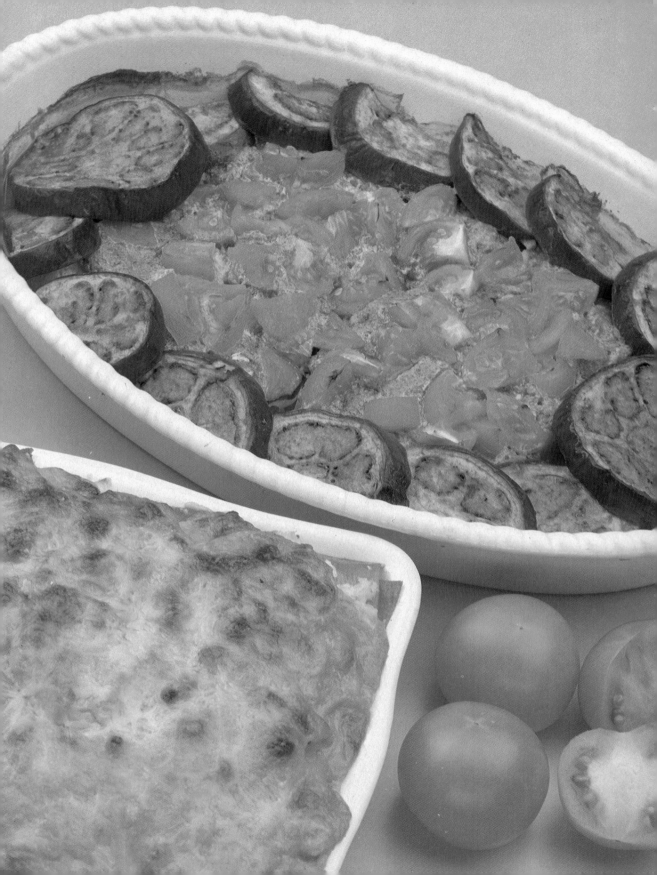

WHITING WITH COURGETTES AND TOMATOES

8 whiting fillets
juice of 1 lemon
450g/1 lb small courgettes
450g/1 lb tomatoes
25g/1 oz butter
1 medium onion, thinly sliced
1 garlic clove, finely chopped
2 tbsp chopped parsley

Skin the fillets and cut crossways into small thin strips. Put the strips on a plate and sprinkle with the lemon juice. Leave to stand for 30 minutes at room temperature. Wipe and thinly slice the courgettes. Scald, skin and thinly slice the tomatoes.

Melt the butter in a large frying pan on a low heat. Stir in the onion and garlic, cover and cook gently for 5 minutes. Add the courgettes, cover again and cook for a further 5 minutes. Uncover the pan and raise the heat to moderate. Carefully mix in the whiting and cook, uncovered, for 2 minutes, gently turning once.

Mix in the tomatoes and let them just heat through.

Transfer everything to a warmed serving dish and scatter the parsley over the top. Serve with brown rice or wholewheat pasta.

KEDGEREE SPECIAL

275g/10 oz long grain brown rice
675g/1½ lb smoked cod or haddock
1 tsp black peppercorns
1 bayleaf
1 slice onion
2 green peppers
4 tbsp oil
1 large onion, thinly sliced
100g/4 oz peanuts
50g/2 oz raisins
2 tsp curry powder
1 tsp ground turmeric
150ml/¼ pint soured cream

Cook the rice in boiling lightly salted water for about 45 minutes until tender. Drain, run cold water through the rice and drain again. Put the cod or haddock into a saucepan with the peppercorns, bayleaf and onion slice. Cover with cold water and bring to the boil. Simmer gently for 2 minutes. Lift out the fish, skin, remove any bones and flake. Core and seed the peppers and cut into 2.5cm/1in strips.

Heat the oil in a large frying pan on a low heat. Put in the peppers and onion and cook until the onion is soft. Mix in the rice, fish, peanuts, raisins, curry powder and turmeric and stir until well heated through.

Put the kedgeree onto a flat serving dish and spoon the soured cream down the centre.

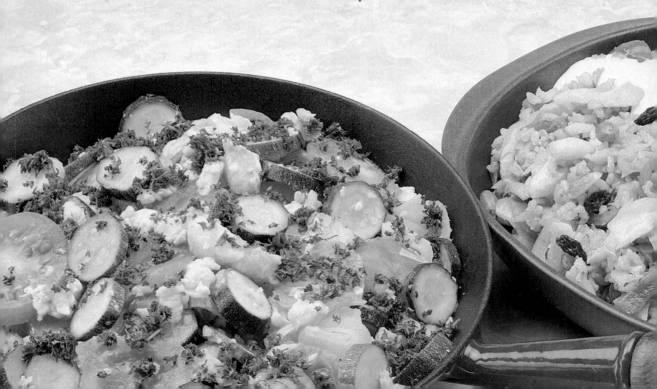

WHITE FISH AND HARICOT BEAN CHOWDER

575g/1¼ lb cod or haddock
100g/4 oz haricot beans, soaked
1.2 litres/2 pints water
1 large onion, thinly sliced
1 slice lemon
2 tbsp oil
bouquet garni
1 bayleaf
25g/1 oz butter
3 tbsp flour
one 350-g/12-oz tin sweetcorn, drained
juice of ½ lemon
sea salt
freshly ground black pepper
6 tbsp chopped parsley

Skin the cod or haddock. Put the fish skin into a saucepan with the beans, water, onion, lemon slice, oil, bouquet garni and bayleaf. Bring to the boil. Cover and simmer for 1 hour 30 minutes or until the beans are soft. Discard the lemon slice, bouquet garni and bayleaf. Work the rest in a blender or food processor until smooth.

Cut the fish into 1cm/½in cubes. Melt the butter in a saucepan on a medium heat. Stir in the flour and the blended soup. Bring to the boil, stirring. Add the fish, sweetcorn, lemon juice and seasonings. Simmer gently for 10 minutes. Add the parsley just before serving.

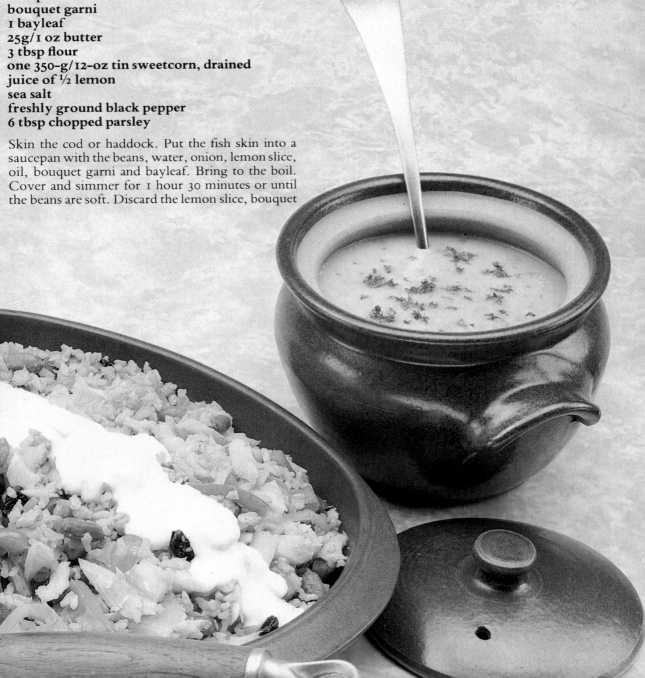

SMOKED MACKEREL AND RICE SALAD

225g/8 oz long grain brown rice
4 tbsp oil
juice of ½ lemon
¼ tsp Tabasco sauce
1 tbsp tomato purée
350g/12 oz smoked mackerel fillets
2 large pickled gherkins
350g/12 oz tomatoes
4 tbsp chopped parsley

Cook the rice in boiling lightly salted water for about 45 minutes until tender. Drain, run cold water through the rice and drain again. Beat together the oil, lemon juice, Tabasco sauce and tomato purée. Add to the rice. Leave the rice until cold.

Skin, bone and flake the mackerel. Thinly slice the cucumbers and chop half the tomatoes. Add the mackerel, cucumbers and chopped tomatoes to the rice.

Spoon the salad onto a serving plate. Slice the remaining tomatoes and use as a garnish. Scatter the parsley over the top.

HERRING AND DILL SALAD

4 small herrings
1 medium onion, halved and thinly sliced
1 tsp dill seeds
3 tbsp water
3 tbsp cider vinegar
2 medium crisp dessert apples
2 medium beetroot, cooked
6 celery sticks
2 large pickled dill cucumbers
150ml/¼ pint natural yoghurt
freshly ground black pepper

Heat the oven to 180°C/350°F/Gas 4. Fillet the herrings and lay the fillets in a large, flat ovenproof dish, overlapping as little as possible. Lay the onion rings on top and sprinkle in the dill seeds. Pour in the water and vinegar. Cover the dish with foil and cook in the oven for 30 minutes. Let the herrings cool completely, still covered.

Finely chop the apples, beetroot, celery and dill cucumbers. Cut the herrings into 2cm/¾in pieces.

Put them all into a large bowl and add the onions from cooking.

Make the dressing by mixing the juices from the herring dish into the yoghurt. Season with pepper to taste. Fold the dressing into the salad.

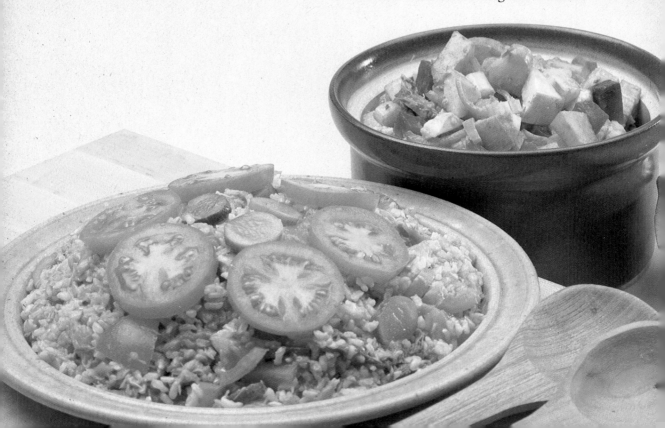

BURGHUL AND TUNA FISH SALAD

225g/ 8 oz burghul wheat (p.48)
1.2 litres/2 pints warm water
one 200-g/7-oz tin tuna fish
12 black olives
6 tbsp olive oil
juice of 1 lemon
1 garlic clove, crushed with a pinch of sea salt
freshly ground black pepper
4 tbsp chopped parsley
2 ripe avocados
4 hard-boiled eggs
½ cucumber
350g/12 oz tomatoes

Soak the wheat in the warm water for 45 minutes. Drain and squeeze dry. Flake the fish with its oil. Halve and stone the olives. Beat together the oil, lemon juice, garlic and pepper. Mix this dressing into the wheat and then fork in the fish, olives and parsley. Spoon the salad into the centre of a serving dish.

Peel and stone the avocados. Halve them crossways and cut the halves into thin strips. Cut the eggs into quarters. Thinly slice the cucumber and cut the tomatoes into wedges. Garnish the salad with the avocados, eggs, cucumber and tomatoes.

MARINATED KIPPER AND CHICORY SALAD

675g/1½ lb kipper fillets
150ml/¼ pint dry white wine
4 tbsp olive oil
1 tbsp tomato purée
8 green olives
1 tbsp chopped thyme
3 heads chicory

Skin the kipper fillets and cut into 1cm/½in strips. Mix together the wine, oil and tomato purée. Stone and chop the olives and add to the marinade with the thyme. Turn the kippers in the marinade, cover and leave for at least 12 hours, at room temperature.

Chop the chicory and mix it into the kippers. Leave the salad for 30 minutes.

Serve with brown bread and butter or a salad of brown rice tossed in French dressing.

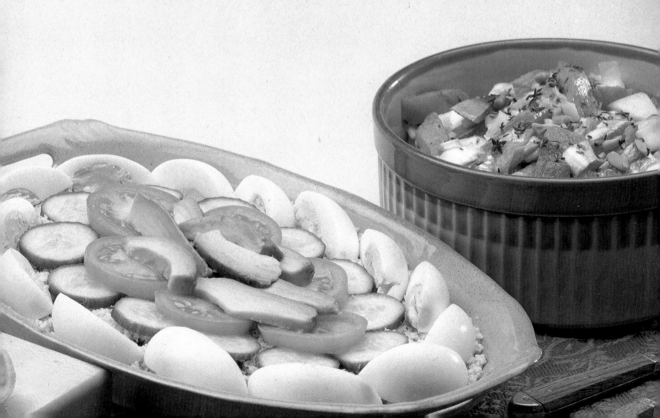

MEAT

Meat, like fish, contains no fibre, but it can be very successfully combined with vegetables, pulses and grains to make high-fibre hot dishes and salads.

MINCED BEEF AND CARROTS

450g/1 lb minced beef
450g/1 lb carrots
2 medium onions, finely chopped
300ml/½ pint stock
1 tbsp chopped thyme
2 tbsp chopped parsley
2 tbsp Worcestershire sauce
sea salt
freshly ground black pepper

Grate the carrots coarsely. Heat a wide-based, flameproof casserole on a high heat with no fat. Put in the minced beef and break it up well. Stir until the beef begins to brown. Mix in the onions, lower the heat and continue cooking, stirring frequently for 2 minutes. Mix in the carrots. Pour in the stock and bring to the boil. Add the herbs and Worcestershire sauce and seasonings.

Cover the casserole and keep on a low heat for 30 minutes.

BEEF, RICE AND RED PEPPERS

675g/1½ lb braising steak or skirt
25g/1 oz butter
2 medium onions, finely chopped
1 garlic clove, finely chopped
2 tsp paprika
½ tsp cayenne pepper
225g/8 oz long grain brown rice
1.2 litres/2 pints stock
2 large red peppers, cored, seeded and chopped
4 tbsp chopped parsley
1 bayleaf

Heat the oven to 160°C/325°F/Gas 3. Cut the beef into 2cm/¾in cubes. Melt the butter in a casserole on a high heat. Put in the beef and brown it well.

Remove the beef and lower the heat. Stir in the onions, garlic, paprika and cayenne pepper and cook until the onions are soft. Stir in the rice and cook for 1 minute. Pour in the stock and bring to the boil. Put in the peppers, parsley and bayleaf and replace the beef.

Cover the casserole and cook in the oven for 1 hour 30 minutes.

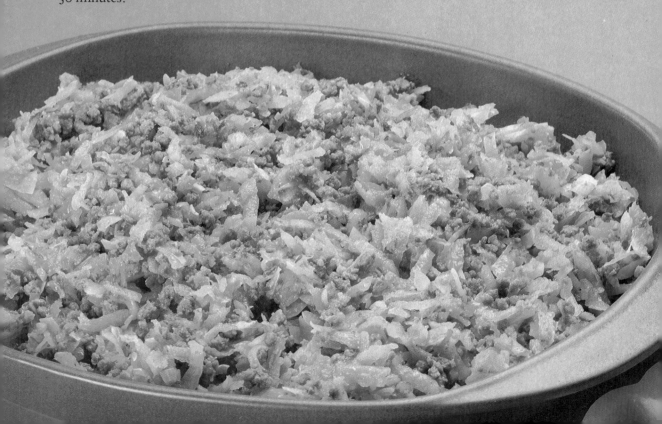

BEEF AND CHICKPEA CURRY

450g/1 lb stewing beef
100g/4 oz chickpeas, soaked and cooked
for 1 hour
350g/12 oz aubergines
1 large green pepper
4 tbsp oil
1 large onion, thinly sliced
1 garlic clove, finely chopped
1 tbsp curry powder
2 tsp paprika
300ml/½ pint stock
1 bayleaf

Heat the oven to 160°C/325°F/Gas 3. Cut the beef into 2.5cm/1in cubes. Dice the aubergines and cut the pepper into 2.5cm/1in strips.

Heat the oil in a flameproof casserole on a high heat. Put in the beef, brown it and remove. Lower the heat. Put in the onion and garlic and cook until soft. Stir in the aubergines, pepper, chickpeas, curry powder and paprika and cook, stirring for 1 minute. Pour in the stock and bring to the boil. Tuck in the bayleaf. Cover the casserole and cook in the oven for 2 hours 15 minutes.

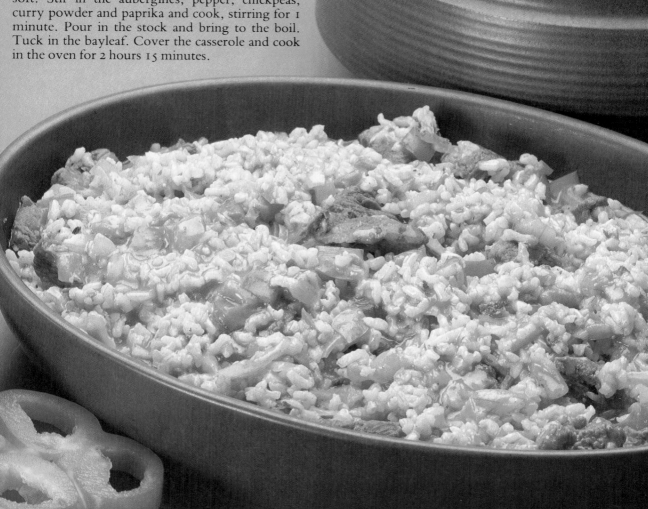

IRISH STEW

675-g/1½-lb neck of lamb
675g/1½ lb potatoes
350g/12 oz carrots
1 small head celery
2 tbsp chopped celery leaves
4 tbsp chopped parsley
sea salt
freshly ground black pepper
600ml/1 pint stock

Ask your butcher to cut the lamb into small chops. Scrub and dice the potatoes. Slice the carrots and chop the celery. Layer the vegetables and meat in a large, flameproof casserole, scattering in the celery leaves and parsley and seasoning to taste as you go.

Pour in the stock. Set the casserole on a medium heat and bring the stock to the boil. Cover, lower the heat and cook gently for 1 hour 30 minutes.

LAMB IN THE BARLEY

½ shoulder of lamb
1.2 litres/2 pints stock
225g/8 oz pot barley (p.48)
sea salt
freshly ground black pepper
bouquet garni
1 bayleaf
225g/8 oz carrots, sliced
4 celery sticks, chopped
1 large onion, thinly sliced

Heat the oven to 180°C/350°F/Gas 4. Heat the grill to high. Lay the lamb on the hot rack and grill until brown on both sides.

Put the stock into a large, flameproof casserole and bring it to the boil. Season and put in the barley, bouquet garni, bayleaf and vegetables. Put the lamb on top. Cover the casserole and cook in the oven for 1 hour 30 minutes.

Carve the lamb and serve it on a bed of barley and vegetables.

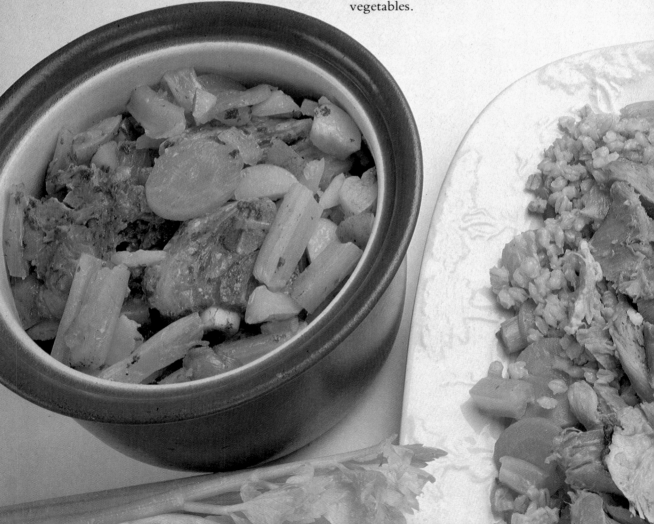

STIR-FRIED SPANISH PORK AND PEAS

900g/2 lb belly pork rashers
200ml/7 fl oz dry white wine
2 tsp ground paprika
¼ tsp cayenne pepper
1 garlic clove, crushed with a pinch of sea salt
900g/2 lb peas (unshelled weight)
15g/½ oz lard
4 tsp chopped chervil or parsley

Cut the rind from the pork rashers. Cut the rashers into pieces about 7.5cm/3in long. Mix the wine, paprika, cayenne pepper and garlic in a dish and add the pieces of pork. Leave to marinate for at least 6 hours at room temperature.

Remove the pork and dice it. Reserve the marinade. Shell the peas. In a large frying pan or wok, heat the lard on a high heat. Put in the pork and stir around until it browns. Lower the heat. Pour off all the fat from the pan. Add the peas. Pour in the marinade and bring to the boil. Add the chervil or parsley. Cover the pan and simmer the pork and peas for 10 minutes.

Serve with brown rice or boiled potatoes.

★ *450g/1 lb frozen peas may be used instead of fresh peas.*

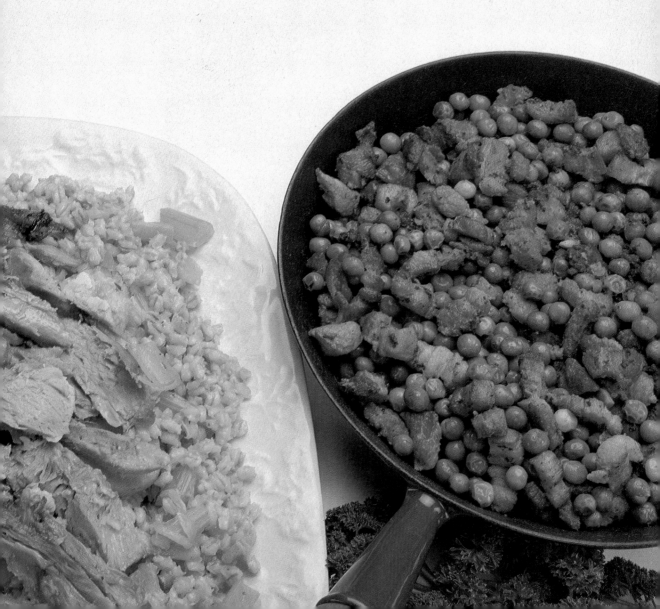

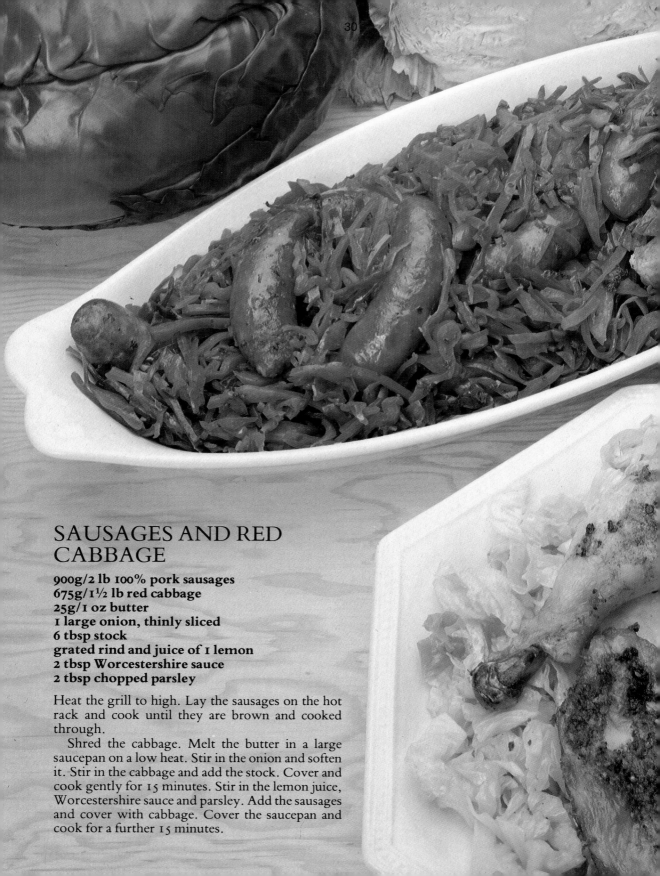

SAUSAGES AND RED CABBAGE

900g/2 lb 100% pork sausages
675g/1½ lb red cabbage
25g/1 oz butter
1 large onion, thinly sliced
6 tbsp stock
grated rind and juice of 1 lemon
2 tbsp Worcestershire sauce
2 tbsp chopped parsley

Heat the grill to high. Lay the sausages on the hot rack and cook until they are brown and cooked through.

Shred the cabbage. Melt the butter in a large saucepan on a low heat. Stir in the onion and soften it. Stir in the cabbage and add the stock. Cover and cook gently for 15 minutes. Stir in the lemon juice, Worcestershire sauce and parsley. Add the sausages and cover with cabbage. Cover the saucepan and cook for a further 15 minutes.

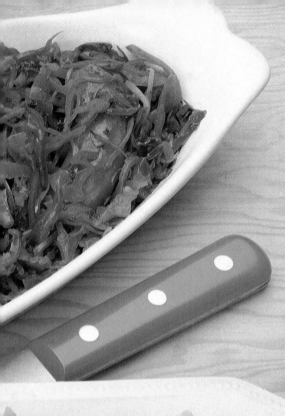

SPICED CHICKEN AND GREEN CABBAGE

one 1.575-kg/3½-lb roasting chicken
6 black peppercorns
6 allspice berries
6 juniper berries
pinch of sea salt
1 garlic clove, finely chopped
25g/1 oz butter, softened
1 large green cabbage

Heat the oven to 200°C/400°F/Gas 6. Joint the chicken and shred the cabbage. Crush together the spices, salt and garlic and mix them into the butter. Spread the spiced butter over the chicken skin. Put the chicken joints into a flameproof casserole, skin-side up. Cook, uncovered, in the oven for 45 minutes or until they are browned and cooked through. Remove and keep warm.

Set the casserole on top of the stove on a medium heat. Stir in the cabbage. Cover the casserole, lower the heat and cook the cabbage for 15 minutes.

Serve the chicken on a bed of cabbage.

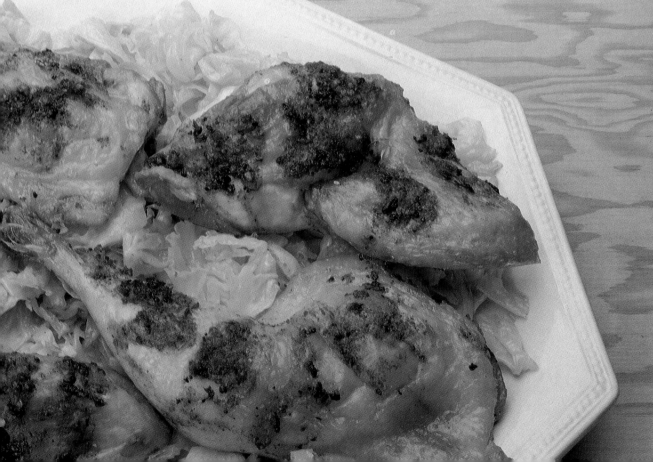

EGGS AND CHEESE

To make fibre-rich meals from eggs and cheese, you have to combine them with other foods that are high in fibre. The simplest way is to make egg and cheese sandwiches with wholewheat bread or serve them on toast. You can also fill omelettes with vegetables, make egg and cheese salads, make a savoury bread pudding or combine eggs and cheese with whole grains and wholewheat pastas.

FRENCH BEAN AND MUSHROOM OMELETTES

225g/8 oz French beans
225g/8 oz button mushrooms
75g/3 oz butter
8 eggs
4 tbsp chopped chervil or parsley
100g/4 oz grated Cheddar cheese

Cook the French beans in the minimum amount of water until they are just tender. Drain and chop into 1cm/½in pieces.

Thinly slice the mushrooms. Melt 25g/1 oz butter in a saucepan on a low heat. Stir in the mushrooms, cover and cook gently for 3 minutes. Remove from the heat and fold in the beans.

Beat 2 eggs with 1 tbsp chervil for each omelette. Melt 15g/½ oz butter in an omelette pan on a high heat. Pour in 2 of the beaten eggs and stir the mixture round with a fork, tipping the pan to ensure the whole base is covered evenly. When the omelette is just set, spoon a quarter of the mushrooms and beans and a quarter of the cheese on one side. Fold over the other half and slide the omelette onto a plate.

Cook the remaining omelettes in the same way.

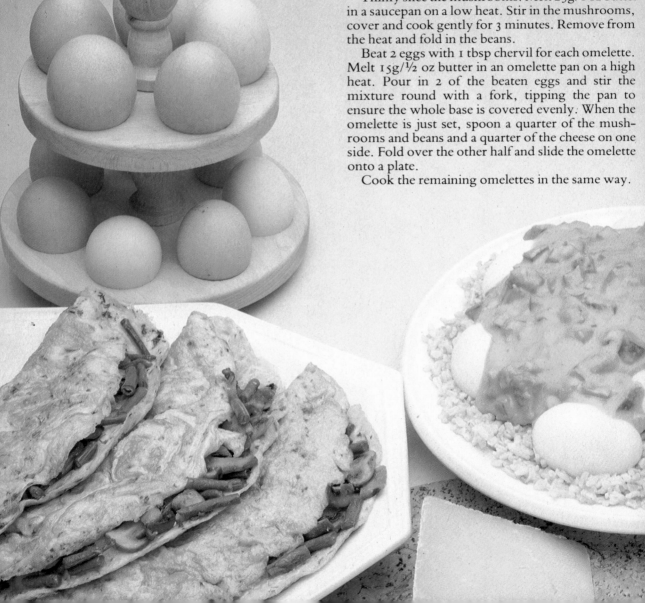

RED HOT EGGS

225g/8 oz long grain brown rice
8 eggs
4 red chillies *or* **¼ tsp cayenne pepper**
2 medium green peppers
50g/2 oz butter
2 tsp paprika
3 tbsp flour
2 tbsp tomato purée
600ml/1 pint milk
2 tbsp chopped parsley

Cook the rice in boiling lightly salted water until tender – about 45 minutes. Drain, rinse with hot water and drain again. Hard boil the eggs. Core, de-seed and finely chop the chillies and peppers.

Melt the butter in a saucepan on a low heat. Stir in the chillies and peppers and cook for 5 minutes. Stir in the paprika (and cayenne pepper if you are using this) and cook for 5 minutes more.

Stir in the flour and cook for 30 seconds. Stir in the tomato purée. Remove the pan from the heat and stir in the milk. Bring the sauce to the boil, stirring all the time, and simmer until the sauce is thick.

Put a bed of rice on a flat serving dish. Peel the eggs, cut in half lengthways and arrange on top of the rice. Pour the sauce over the eggs and garnish with the parsley.

EGGS IN POTATOES

4 large baking potatoes
25g/1 oz butter
100g/4 oz grated Double Gloucester cheese
8 spring onions, finely chopped
2 tbsp chopped parsley
sea salt
freshly ground black pepper
8 small eggs

Heat the oven to 200°C/400°F/Gas 6. Scrub the potatoes and prick each one 4 times with a fork. Bake the potatoes on the oven rack for 1 hour 30 minutes. Cut in half lengthways and scoop all the flesh into a bowl. Mash with half the cheese and all the butter, onions and parsley. Season.

Line each potato shell with a very thin layer of mashed potato mixture and put the shells on a large, flat, heatproof serving dish. Arrange the rest of the mashed potato round them. Break an egg into each shell.

Sprinkle the remaining cheese over the eggs. Cook in the oven for 30 minutes so the eggs are set and the surrounding potato is golden brown.

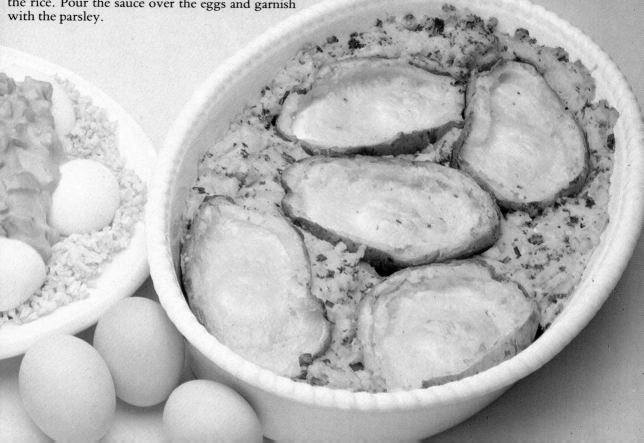

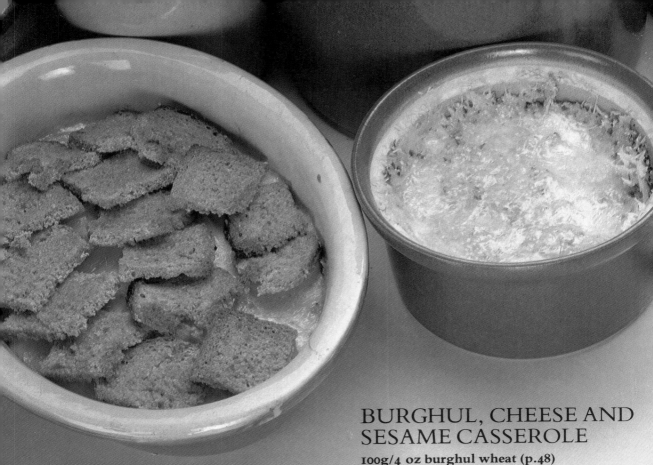

CRISPY CHESHIRE CHEESE AND TOMATO BAKE

8 slices wholewheat bread
450g/1 lb tomatoes
225g/8 oz grated Cheshire cheese
3 eggs
200ml/7 fl oz milk
2 tsp made English mustard
butter

Heat the oven to 200°C/400°F/Gas 6. Dice half the bread and put in the base of a large pie dish. Slice the tomatoes into rounds and lay half on top of the breadcubes.

Beat the cheese, eggs, milk and mustard together and pour the mixture evenly over the tomatoes.

Arrange the remaining tomatoes on top of the cheese mixture. Thickly butter the remaining bread. Cut the slices into fairly large squares and lay them over the tomatoes.

Bake for 30 minutes and serve hot.

BURGHUL, CHEESE AND SESAME CASSEROLE

100g/4 oz burghul wheat (p.48)
675g/1½ lb tomatoes
20 green olives
2 red peppers
4 tbsp olive oil
2 large onions, quartered and thinly sliced
1 garlic clove, finely chopped
225g/8 oz grated Cheddar cheese
4 tbsp sesame seeds
2 tbsp chopped parsley
1 tbsp chopped thyme

Heat the oven to 200°C/400°F/Gas 6. Soak the wheat in warm water for 20 minutes. Drain the wheat and squeeze dry. Scald and skin the tomatoes and cut into crossways slices.

Stone and quarter the olives. Core and seed the peppers and cut into 2.5cm/1in strips. Heat the oil in a frying pan on a low heat. Mix in the onions, garlic and peppers. Cook until the onions are soft and remove from the heat.

Put a quarter of the onions and peppers in the bottom of a casserole, then a quarter of the tomatoes, the olives and the same of the wheat, sesame seeds, herbs and cheese. Make three more layers in the same way. Cover the casserole and cook in the oven for 30 minutes.

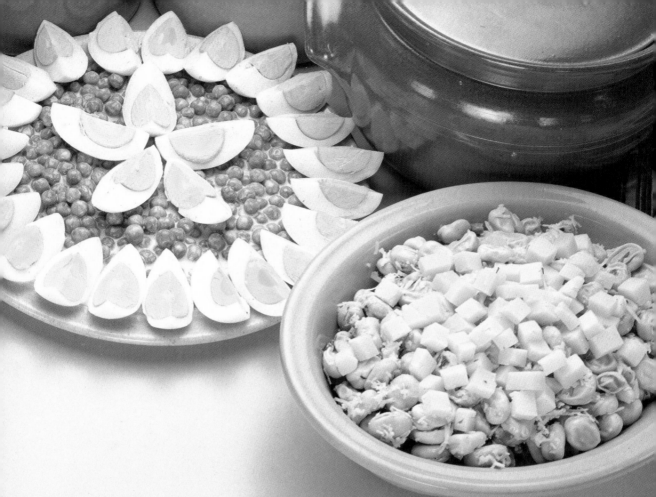

PEA AND EGG SALAD

8 eggs
900g/2 lb peas (unshelled weight)
200ml/7 fl oz stock (preferably ham)

DRESSING
1 egg yolk
1 tsp Dijon mustard
6 tbsp oil
6 tbsp natural yoghurt

Hard boil and cool the eggs. Shell the peas. Bring the stock to the boil, put in the peas and simmer for 15 minutes. Drain.

To make the dressing, beat the egg yolk with the mustard. Beat in the oil drop by drop and then beat in the yoghurt by the tablespoon. Fold the peas into the dressing while they are still warm and leave until they are completely cold.

Shell the eggs and cut into quarters. Arrange the peas in the centre of a serving plate with the eggs round the edge.

★ 450g/1 lb frozen peas may be used instead of fresh peas.

BROAD BEAN AND CHEESE SALAD

1.8kg/4 lb broad beans
125ml/4 fl oz olive oil
8 spring onions, finely chopped
2 tbsp chopped savory
4 tbsp cider vinegar
175g/6 oz Cheddar cheese

Shell the beans. Heat the oil in a saucepan on a low heat. Stir in the beans, onions and savory. Cover and cook gently for 20 minutes, stirring occasionally. The beans should be just cooked.

Take the pan from the heat and mix in the cider vinegar. Leave until the beans are completely cold.

Just before serving, finely grate 100g/4 oz of cheese and fold into the beans. Dice the rest and scatter over the top.

★ 900g/2 lb frozen broad beans may be used instead of fresh beans.

SWEETCORN, EGG AND BACON PIE

4 eggs
one 350–g/12–oz tin sweetcorn
225g/8 oz lean bacon
1 red pepper
1 green pepper
15g/½ oz butter
1 large onion, finely chopped
1 garlic clove, finely chopped
2 tbsp wholewheat flour
200ml/7 fl oz stock
1 tbsp tomato purée
1 tsp paprika
pinch cayenne pepper
2 tsp chopped thyme
1 tbsp chopped parsley
shortcrust pastry made with
    350g/12 oz wholewheat flour
beaten egg for glaze

Heat the oven to 200°C/400°F/Gas 6. Hard boil and chop the eggs. Drain the sweetcorn. Chop the bacon. Core, seed and dice the peppers.

Melt the butter in a saucepan on a low heat. Put in the bacon, peppers, onion and garlic and cook until the onion is soft and the bacon cooked but not coloured.

Stir in the flour and then the stock. Bring to the boil, stirring. Add the tomato purée, paprika, cayenne pepper and herbs and simmer for 2 minutes. Take the pan from the heat and stir in the sweetcorn and eggs.

Roll out about two-thirds of the pastry and line a 25cm/10in flan tin. Put in the filling and cover with the remaining rolled-out pastry. Seal the edges and brush the top with beaten egg. Bake the pie for 30 minutes or until golden brown. Serve hot.

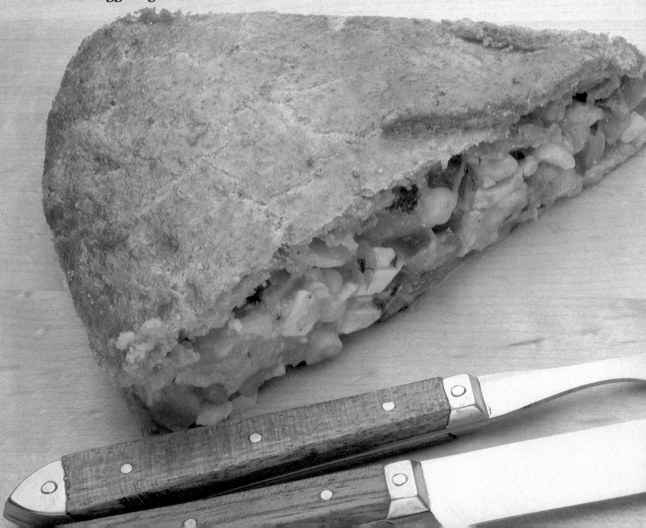

CELERY, POTATO AND CHEESE PIE

6 celery sticks
450g/1 lb potatoes
25g/1 oz butter
1 large onion, thinly sliced
2 tbsp wholewheat flour
300ml/½ pint milk
3 tbsp chopped parsley
1 garlic clove, crushed with a pinch of sea salt
pinch cayenne pepper
75g/3 oz grated Cheddar cheese
75g/3 oz grated blue cheese
shortcrust pastry made with
    350g/12 oz wholewheat flour
beaten egg for glaze

Heat the oven to 200°C/400°F/Gas 6. Chop the celery. Scrub and thinly slice the potatoes. Steam the celery and potatoes together for 20 minutes so they are just tender.

Melt the butter in a saucepan on a moderate heat. Add the onion and cook until soft. Stir in the flour and milk and bring to the boil, stirring. Simmer the sauce for 2 minutes. Take the pan from the heat and beat in the parsley, garlic, cayenne pepper and cheeses. Fold in the celery and potatoes and cool the mixture slightly.

Roll out about two-thirds of the pastry and line a 25cm/10in flan tin. Put in the filling and cover with the remaining rolled-out pastry. Seal the edges and brush the top with beaten egg. Bake the pie for 30 minutes or until golden brown. Serve hot.

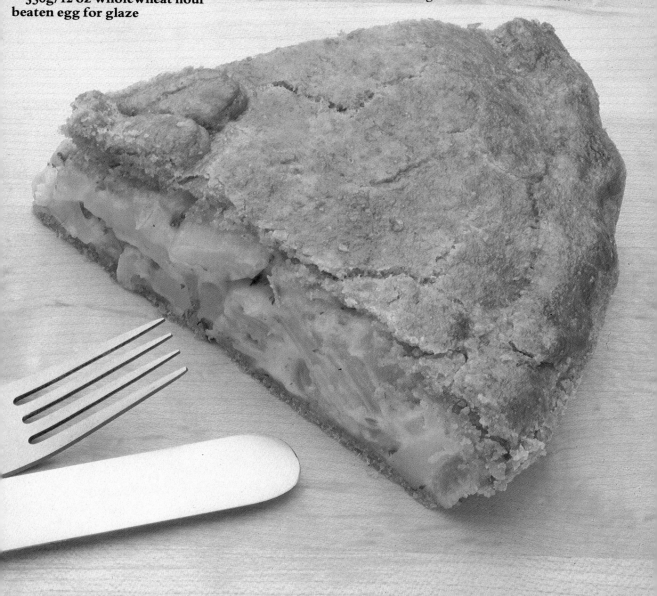

PULSES AND NUTS

The pulse vegetables, dried beans and lentils, are some of the most fibre-rich foods. Nuts contain some fibre and as they are often mixed with vegetables and whole grains in savoury vegetarian dishes, the fibre content of nut meals is generally high.

Dried beans need to be soaked before they are cooked. Either soak them overnight in cold water or use the quick method. Put the beans into a saucepan with cold water, bring to the boil, boil for 2 minutes and then leave in the same water to soak for between 1 hour 30 minutes and 2 hours.

Beans must be properly cooked to make them pleasant to eat and also to drive away any harmful substances that may cause slight illness. These harmful substances are only found in kidney beans, flageolets, haricot beans and aduki beans, but if all beans are given the same cooking method it is easier to remember the procedure. Bring the beans to the boil in their soaking water, boil for 15 minutes and drain. Then return the beans to the saucepan with fresh water and simmer until tender. Black-eyed beans and mung beans take 45 minutes, aduki beans 1 hour, haricot beans, flageolets and kidney beans 1 hour 30 minutes, butter beans 2 hours and chick-peas and soya beans up to 3 hours.

Lentils need no soaking and most take 45 minutes to cook. In order to provide a well-balanced protein meal, unless the dish also contains meat, fish, eggs or cheese, dried beans and lentils should be served with whole grains such as wholewheat bread or toast, brown rice, cooked wheat or barley grains, burghul wheat or wholewheat pasta.

AUBERGINE AND HARICOT BEAN CASSEROLE

225g/8 oz haricot beans, soaked and cooked
2 large aubergines
1 tbsp sea salt
450g/1 lb tomatoes
4 tbsp olive oil
1 large onion, quartered and thinly sliced
1 garlic clove, finely chopped
2 tsp paprika
¼ tsp cayenne pepper
150ml/¼ pint dry white wine
1 tbsp chopped thyme
1 tbsp chopped parsley
175g/6 oz Mozarella cheese
1 tbsp Dijon mustard

Heat the oven to 200°C/400°F/Gas 6. Cut the aubergines into 2cm/¾in dice, put in a colander and sprinkle with the salt. Leave for 30 minutes to drain. Rinse with cold water and pat dry with kitchen paper. Scald, skin and chop the tomatoes.

Heat the oil in a frying pan on a low heat. Mix in the onion and garlic and cook until they are soft. Add the aubergines and cook for 2 minutes. Mix in

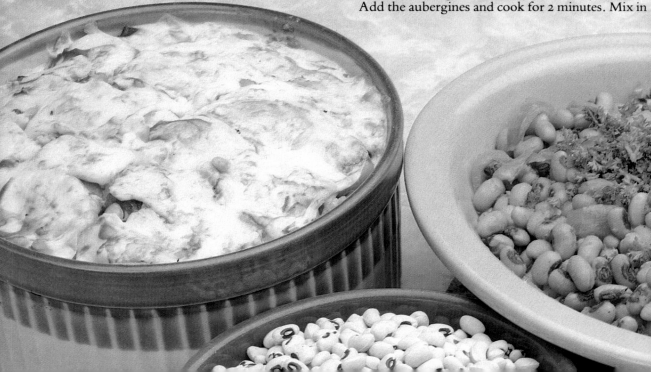

the paprika, cayenne pepper and tomatoes. Pour in the wine and bring to the boil.

Add the herbs and mix in the beans. Transfer everything to a deep ovenproof dish. Cover the dish with foil and cook in the oven for 45 minutes.

Cut the cheese into thin slices. Remove the foil from the dish, lay the slices of cheese over the beans and spread with the mustard. Put the dish back into the oven, uncovered, for 10 minutes so the cheese melts and begins to brown. Serve straight from the dish.

★ Stock may be used instead of wine. The cheese may be omitted if wished.

SPICED BLACK-EYED BEANS

225g/8 oz black-eyed beans, soaked and cooked
600ml/1 pint water
4 tbsp oil
1 large onion, quartered and thinly sliced
1 large garlic clove, finely chopped
1 tsp ground mixed spice
1 tsp paprika
150ml/¼ pint stock
2 tbsp tomato purée
2 tbsp chopped fresh coriander or parsley

Heat the oil in a saucepan on a low heat. Mix in the onion, garlic, mixed spice and paprika and cook until the onion is soft. Stir in the beans, stock and tomato purée. Cover and keep on a very low heat for 10 minutes.

Serve with brown rice or cooked burghul wheat.

RED BEANS AND PASTA

225g/8 oz red beans, soaked and cooked
300g/11 oz small pasta shapes
3 tbsp olive oil
2 medium onions, thinly sliced
1 garlic clove, finely chopped
450g/1 lb tomatoes, scalded, skinned and chopped
2 tbsp chopped basil
3 tbsp chopped parsley
100g/4 oz grated Gruyère or Cheddar cheese (optional)

Boil the pasta shapes in lightly salted water for about 10–15 minutes until tender. Drain and rinse through with hot water.

While the pasta is cooking, heat the oil in a saucepan on a low heat. Put in the onions and garlic and cook until soft. Add the tomatoes and herbs and cook gently, uncovered, for 3 minutes, so the tomatoes soften.

Mix in the beans and pasta and heat them through. Turn onto a warmed serving dish and scatter the cheese over the top.

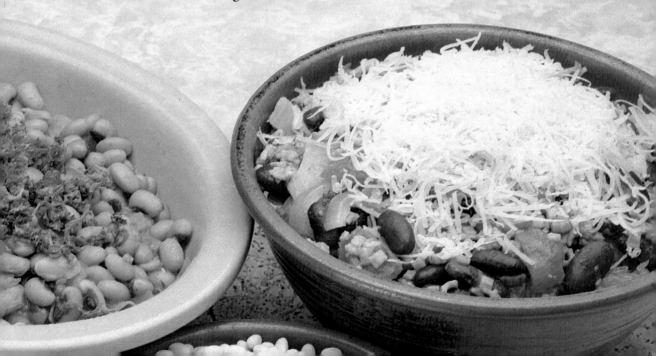

YELLOW PEAS AND SPICED SAUSAGE

225g/8 oz spiced continental sausage
2 medium onions, quartered and thinly sliced
1 garlic clove, finely chopped
225g/8 oz yellow split peas
1 tbsp paprika
600ml/1 pint ham stock
1 bayleaf

Thinly slice the sausage. Put the sausage slices into a saucepan and set on a low heat. When the fat begins to run, in about 1 minute, add the onions and garlic and cook until soft.

Stir in the peas and paprika and continue stirring for 1 minute. Pour in the stock and bring to the boil. Add the bayleaf.

Cover and simmer for 45 minutes, beating towards the end so the peas make a thick purée. Remove the bayleaf before serving.

★ *Chorizo, Mettwurst and Katsanos are all suitable types of sausage to use. If none of these is available, use a boiling sausage and add 15g/½ oz butter or 2 tbsp oil when cooking.*

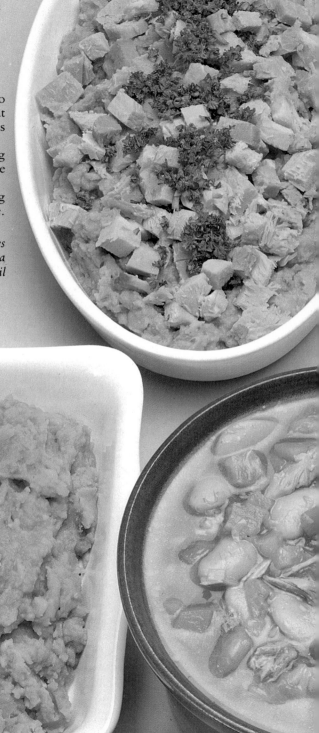

GREEN PEA PURÉE WITH BACON

1 fore-knuckle bacon joint weighing
    about 675g/1½ lb
1 bayleaf
1 tsp black peppercorns
4 cloves
225g/8 oz green split peas
4 large celery sticks
2 medium carrots
1 medium onion
freshly ground black pepper
bouquet garni
2 tbsp chopped parsley

Soak the bacon overnight, or bring to the boil, drain, rinse in cold water and drain again. Put the joint into a large saucepan and cover with fresh water. Add the bayleaf, peppercorns and cloves and bring to the boil on a moderate heat. Cover and simmer for 1 hour.

Lift out the bacon and cut away the rind. Strain and reserve the stock. Finely chop the celery, carrots and onion. Put them into the rinsed-out saucepan with the bacon and peas. Pour in 600ml/ 1 pint of the stock and season well with pepper. Add the bouquet garni. Bring everything to the boil again and simmer, covered, for 1 hour so the

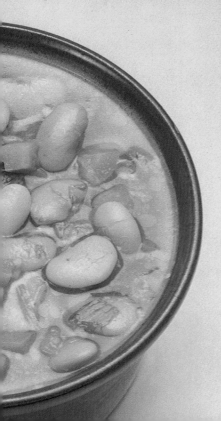

peas are reduced to a soft purée. If there is still any stock in the saucepan, simmer the peas until it is absorbed.

Lift out the bacon and dice. Arrange the pea purée on a warmed serving dish. Place the ham on top and sprinkle with the parsley.

Serve with jacket potatoes and no other vegetables – but have a salad for a first course.

CHICKEN AND BUTTER BEAN SOUP

1 chicken carcass
2 chicken wing tips
1 set chicken giblets, excluding liver
BOILING
3.6 litres/6 pints water
1 onion, cut in half, not peeled
1 carrot, roughly chopped
1 celery stick, roughly chopped
1 tsp black peppercorns
bouquet garni

SOUP
225g/8 oz butter beans, soaked and cooked
    for 1 hour
450g/1 lb leeks, thinly sliced
450g/1 lb carrots, finely chopped
225g/8 oz celery, finely chopped
bouquet garni
sea salt
freshly ground black pepper
4 tbsp chopped parsley

Put the chicken pieces into a large saucepan with the boiling ingredients. Bring to the boil and skim. Cover and simmer for 1 hour 30 minutes.

Strain the stock from the chicken, and reserve it. Discard the vegetables. Scrape all the meat from the chicken carcass and the neck. Finely chop the heart. Discard the rest.

Bring the reserved stock to the boil. Put in the butter beans, leeks, carrots, celery and bouquet garni. Season well. Cover and simmer for 1–2 hours so the butter beans are completely tender.

Take out half the soup and work in a blender or food processor until smooth and thick. Alternatively, rub half the soup through a vegetable mill. Stir it back into the rest.

Add the chicken meat and reheat. Add the parsley and serve in large, deep bowls as a main meal. Accompany it with wholewheat bread and a salad.

★ *This is a good way of utilizing a chicken carcass from which you have taken the joints for another dish. If one is not available, use one or more sets of giblets.*

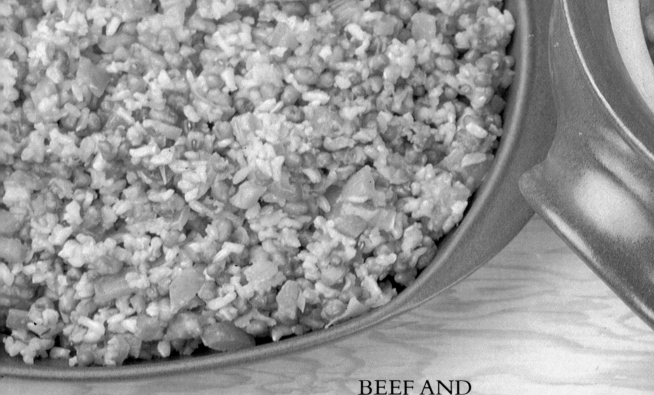

MUNG BEANS AND BROWN RICE

225g/8 oz mung beans, soaked
4 tbsp oil
2 medium onions, finely chopped
1 garlic clove, finely chopped
175g/6 oz carrots, finely chopped
6 celery sticks, finely chopped
225g/8 oz long grain brown rice
600ml/1 pint stock
3 tbsp tamari or soy sauce
¼ tsp sea salt
1 bayleaf

Put the mung beans into a saucepan with fresh water. Bring to the boil, boil for 15 minutes and drain.

Heat the oil in a large saucepan on a low heat. Stir in the onions, garlic, carrots and celery and cook for 4 minutes, stirring occasionally. Stir in the beans and rice. Pour in the stock and bring to the boil. Add the soy sauce, salt and bayleaf. Cover and simmer for 45 minutes or until both rice and beans are tender.

Tamari sauce is a natural soy sauce available from wholefood shops.

BEEF AND SPLIT PEA SOUP

350g/12 oz stewing beef

BOILING
1 onion, cut in half, not peeled
1 large carrot, cut lengthways
1 celery stick, broken into 3 pieces
bouquet garni
1 tsp black peppercorns
¼ tsp ground allspice
½ tsp sea salt
1.8 litres/3 pints water

SOUP
1 large onion, finely chopped
4 large celery sticks, finely chopped
225g/8 oz carrots, finely chopped
225g/8 oz yellow split peas
sea salt
freshly ground black pepper

Put the beef into a saucepan with the boiling ingredients. Bring to the boil, cover and simmer for 1 hour 30 minutes. Strain off the stock. Reserve the beef and discard the vegetables.

Finely shred the beef. Bring the stock to the boil in a clean saucepan. Add the onion, celery, carrots and split peas and season well. Put in the beef, cover and simmer for 1 hour.

Serve as a main meal in large, deep bowls. Accompany it with wholewheat bread and a salad.

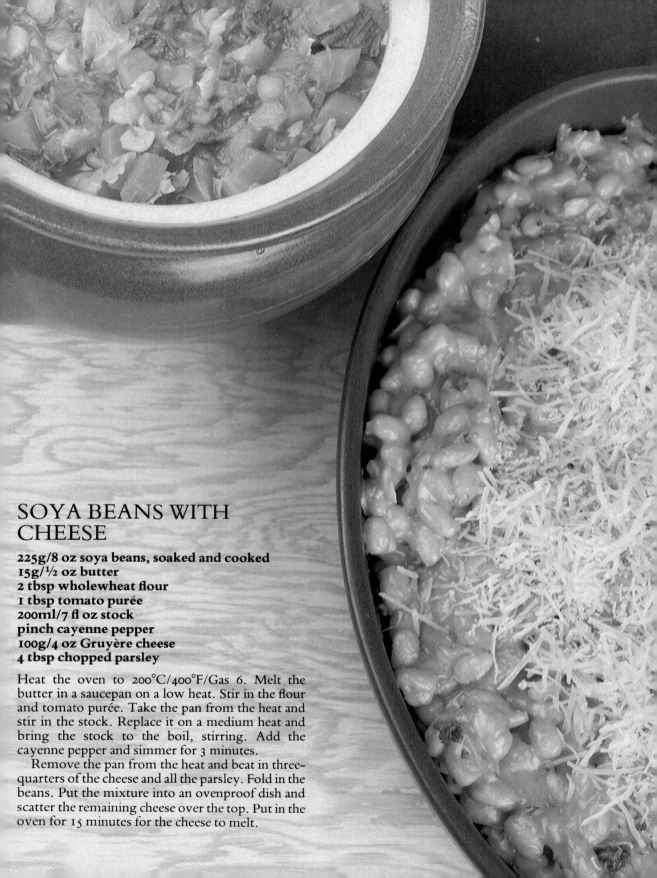

SOYA BEANS WITH CHEESE

225g/8 oz soya beans, soaked and cooked
15g/½ oz butter
2 tbsp wholewheat flour
1 tbsp tomato purée
200ml/7 fl oz stock
pinch cayenne pepper
100g/4 oz Gruyère cheese
4 tbsp chopped parsley

Heat the oven to 200°C/400°F/Gas 6. Melt the butter in a saucepan on a low heat. Stir in the flour and tomato purée. Take the pan from the heat and stir in the stock. Replace it on a medium heat and bring the stock to the boil, stirring. Add the cayenne pepper and simmer for 3 minutes.

Remove the pan from the heat and beat in three-quarters of the cheese and all the parsley. Fold in the beans. Put the mixture into an ovenproof dish and scatter the remaining cheese over the top. Put in the oven for 15 minutes for the cheese to melt.

RED AND GREEN BEAN SALAD

225g/8 oz red kidney beans, soaked and cooked
450g/1 lb French beans
4 tbsp olive oil
2 medium onions, thinly sliced
2 tbsp red wine vinegar
2 tbsp chopped thyme

Cook the French beans in lightly salted simmering water for 10 minutes. Drain and cut into 2.5cm/1in lengths.

Heat the oil in a saucepan on a low heat. Stir in the onions and cook until they are soft. Mix in the kidney beans.

Pour in the vinegar and let it bubble. Take the pan from the heat and fold in the French beans and thyme. Leave the salad until it is completely cool before serving.

★ *The yellow variety of French beans may be used instead of green.*

LENTIL, TOMATO AND CELERY SALAD

225g/8 oz brown or green lentils
bouquet garni
1 bayleaf
4 tbsp sunflower oil
4 tbsp white wine vinegar
2 tbsp tomato purée
2 tsp paprika
½ tsp Tabasco sauce
freshly ground black pepper
8 celery sticks
350g/12 oz tomatoes, sliced

Put the lentils into a saucepan with the bouquet garni and bayleaf. Cover with water, bring to the boil and simmer for 45 minutes or until they are very tender. Drain, and discard the bouquet garni and bayleaf.

Mash the lentils to a purée and work in the oil, vinegar, tomato purée, paprika, Tabasco sauce and pepper. Mix well.

Finely chop the celery and mix into the lentils. Put the salad onto a serving dish and surround with tomato slices.

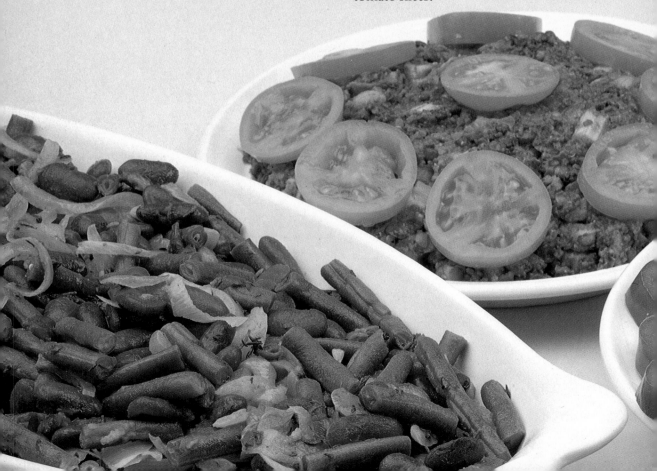

CHICKPEA AND LEMON SALAD

225g/8 oz chickpeas, soaked and cooked
2 lemons
4 tbsp olive oil
2 tbsp tahini
1 garlic clove, crushed with a pinch of sea salt
   or 3 tbsp chopped chives
freshly ground black pepper
2 tbsp sesame seeds
1 large onion, sliced into rings
1 large green pepper
225g/8 oz tomatoes

Put the chickpeas into a bowl. Cut the rind and pith from one of the lemons and finely chop the flesh. Mix into the chickpeas. Squeeze the juice from the remaining lemon and beat with the oil and tahini.

Add the garlic or chives. Season. Fold the dressing into the chickpeas.

Put the chickpeas onto a large, flat serving plate and scatter with the sesame seeds and onion rings. Core and seed the pepper and slice into semi-circles. Thinly slice the tomatoes. Arrange the pepper and tomatoes round the edge of the chickpeas.

★ *Tahini is a paste made from ground sesame seeds that can be bought from wholefood shops.*

BURGHUL, CUCUMBER AND WALNUT SALAD

225g/8 oz burghul wheat (p.48)
1 medium cucumber
100g/4 oz chopped walnuts
4 tbsp chopped dill
4 tbsp olive oil
2 tbsp white wine vinegar
1 garlic clove, crushed with a pinch of sea salt
freshly ground black pepper
1 lettuce

Soak the wheat in cold water for 30 minutes. Drain and squeeze dry. Finely chop the cucumber, reserving 4 slices for garnish.

Put the burghul, cucumber, walnuts and dill into a bowl. Beat the oil, vinegar, garlic and pepper together to make the dressing and fold into the salad. Leave the salad for 15 minutes. Arrange the lettuce leaves on a large serving plate and pile the salad on top.

★ *This makes a light meal in itself. A tomato salad is a good accompaniment.*

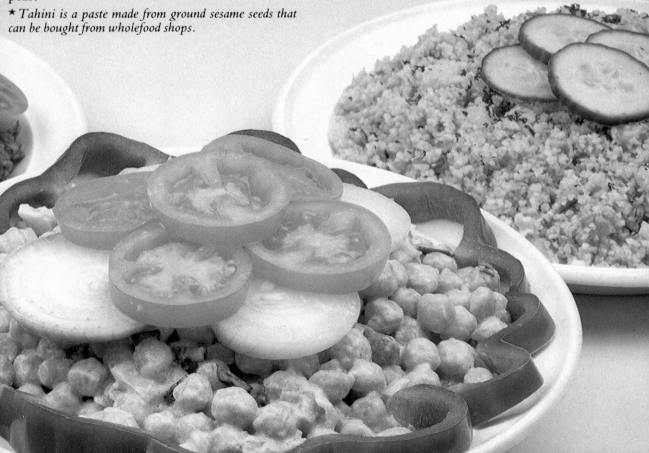

MUESLI, PEANUT AND CARROT SALAD

225g/8 oz muesli base (p.6)
275g/10 oz carrots
175g/6 oz peanuts
50g/2 oz raisins
300ml/½ pint natural yoghurt
2 tbsp tomato purée
1 tsp ground cinnamon
1 garlic clove, crushed with a pinch of sea salt
freshly ground black pepper
1 bunch watercress

Put the muesli into a bowl. Coarsely grate the carrots and mix into the muesli with the peanuts and raisins. Put the yoghurt into a small bowl and beat in the tomato purée, cinnamon, garlic and pepper. Fold into the muesli mixture.

Put the salad onto a serving plate and garnish with watercress sprigs.

★ This makes an all-in-one salad meal.

LENTIL AND HAZELNUT PATTIES

225g/8 oz split red lentils
4 tbsp oil
1 large onion, finely chopped
1 garlic clove, finely chopped
600ml/1 pint stock
1 bayleaf
sea salt
freshly ground black pepper
175g/6 oz shelled hazelnuts, finely chopped
4 tbsp chopped parsley
1 tbsp chopped thyme
2 sage leaves, chopped
2 tbsp tomato purée
50g/2 oz wholewheat flour, seasoned
oil for shallow frying

Heat the oil in a heavy saucepan on a low heat. Stir in the onion and garlic and cook until the onion is soft. Add the lentils and cook for 2 minutes, stirring. Pour in the stock and bring to the boil. Season well and add the bayleaf. Cover and simmer gently for 45 minutes, beating the lentils to a thick purée with a wooden spoon towards the end.

Take the pan from the heat and let the lentils cool, keeping them covered to prevent a hard surface developing. Beat in the hazelnuts, parsley, thyme, sage and tomato purée. Form the mixture into 12 round, flat patties and coat in the seasoned flour.

Shallow fry the patties on a moderate heat until they are golden brown on both sides.

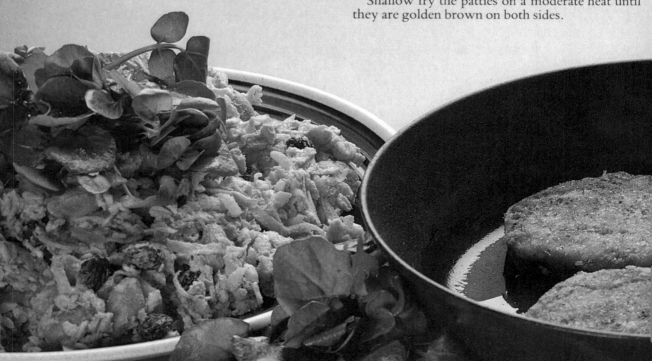

NUT AND WHEAT ROAST

175g/6 oz shelled walnuts
50g/2 oz shelled Brazil nuts
6 tbsp sunflower oil
2 medium onions, chopped
1 garlic clove, chopped
100g/4 oz burghul wheat (p.48)
175ml/6 fl oz dry white wine
3 tbsp tomato purée
2 tbsp chopped parsley
1 tbsp chopped thyme
2 tsp chopped rosemary
6 sage leaves, chopped

Heat the oven to 200°C/400°F/Gas 6. Grind the nuts in a blender or mill. Heat the oil in a frying pan on a low heat. Mix in the onions and garlic and cook for 2 minutes. Stir in the wheat and cook, stirring, for 5 minutes. Pour in the wine, bring to the boil and cook gently for 5 minutes, stirring frequently. Take the pan from the heat and mix in the nuts, tomato purée and herbs. Press the mixture into an ovenproof dish and bake for 40 minutes, or until well browned.

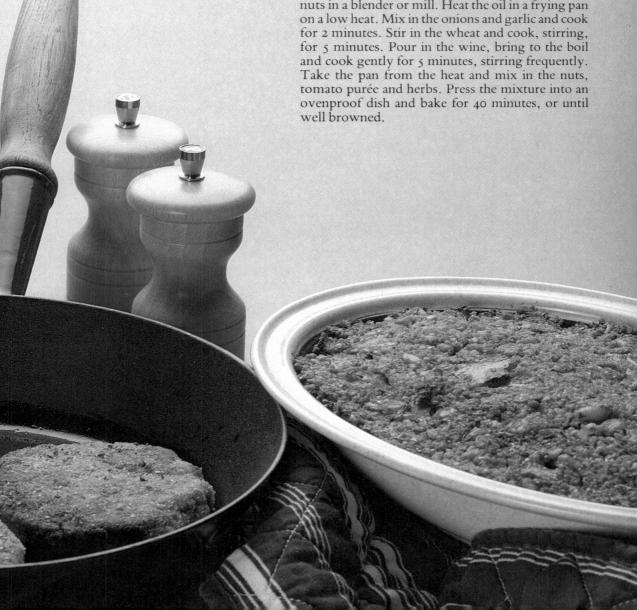

GRAINS AND PASTAS

All grains are extremely high in fibre, provided they remain in their unrefined state and the outer coating of the grain or bran, as it is called, is not removed.

Wholewheat is very often only thought of in terms of wholewheat flour, but the wheat grains themselves can be cooked and served as a savoury accompaniment to a protein dish. Another type of wholewheat called burghul can be bought in wholefood shops. It consists of wheat that has been soaked and cooked at a high temperature so that it cracks into small pieces. It can be served, uncooked, as a salad or cooked as a hot alternative to potatoes or rice.

Brown rice consists of unrefined rice grains that still retain their outer coating of bran. It has a nutty flavour and slightly chewy texture and the grains never stick together when cooked. It does, however, need a long cooking time of 40–45 minutes. There are long grain and short grain varieties. Both can be used to make savoury dishes and the short grain type can be used to make rice puddings.

Instead of pearl barley in casseroles and soups use pot barley which can also be bought from wholefood shops. It can be substituted in most dishes by oat groats which are whole oat grains. Rolled oats and fine, coarse and medium oatmeal are all produced from whole oat grains.

For more unusual dishes choose buckwheat grain which is often made into a dish called kasha, or millet which can be cooked in the same way as burghul.

A wide range of wholewheat pasta is now readily available in most shops. Wholewheat pasta has more flavour than white. It takes about the same amount of time to cook – about 15 minutes – and can be used in exactly the same type of dishes.

STEAMED TURMERIC RICE WITH CURRANTS

225g/8 oz short grain brown rice
3 tbsp olive oil or sunflower oil
1 medium onion, finely chopped
2 tsp ground turmeric
50g/2 oz currants
600ml/1 pint stock
pinch of sea salt

Heat the oil in a saucepan on a low heat. Add the onion and cook until it is soft. Stir in the rice, turmeric and currants and cook for 1 minute, stirring.

Pour in the stock and bring to the boil. Season, cover and simmer for 45 minutes. Turn off the heat and let the rice stand for 10 minutes.

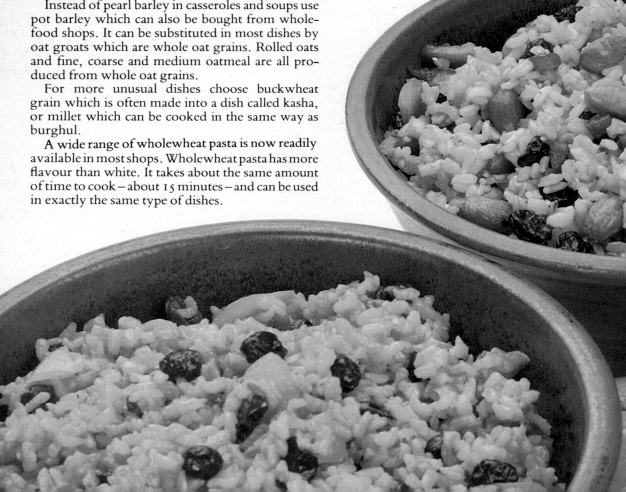

BROWN RICE AND PEANUT SALAD

225g/8 oz brown rice
4 tbsp oil
2 tbsp cider vinegar
1 tbsp tamari sauce
1 garlic clove, crushed with a pinch of sea salt
freshly ground black pepper
100g/4 oz peanuts
1 green pepper, cored, seeded and chopped
50g/2 oz raisins

Cook the rice in lightly salted boiling water for about 45 minutes, or until tender. Drain, rinse with cold water and drain again. Beat together the oil, vinegar, tamari sauce, garlic and pepper. Mix the dressing into the rice. Leave the rice to cool.

Mix in the peanuts, pepper and raisins. Leave the salad for 15 minutes before serving.

RICE AND PORK FRY

275g/10 oz long grain brown rice
225g/8 oz belly pork rashers
100g/4 oz boiling sausage
2 medium oranges
1 large onion, quartered and thinly sliced
1 garlic clove, finely chopped
one 175-g/6-oz tin sweetcorn, drained
1 tsp paprika
¼ tsp cayenne pepper

Cook the rice in lightly salted boiling water for about 45 minutes, or until tender. Drain, rinse with cold water and drain again.

Cut the rind and any bones from the pork. Dice the rashers. Thinly slice the boiling sausage. Cut the rind and pith from the oranges. Cut each orange in half and thinly slice.

Heat a large, heavy frying pan on a high heat with no fat. Put in the pork and stir until it browns. Lower the heat and add the onion, garlic and sliced sausage. Cook until the onion is soft. Mix in the rice and sweetcorn, paprika and cayenne pepper. Stir until the rice has heated through. Mix in the pieces of orange and cook for 1 minute more.

★ *This is a meal in itself, needing only a salad as an accompaniment.*

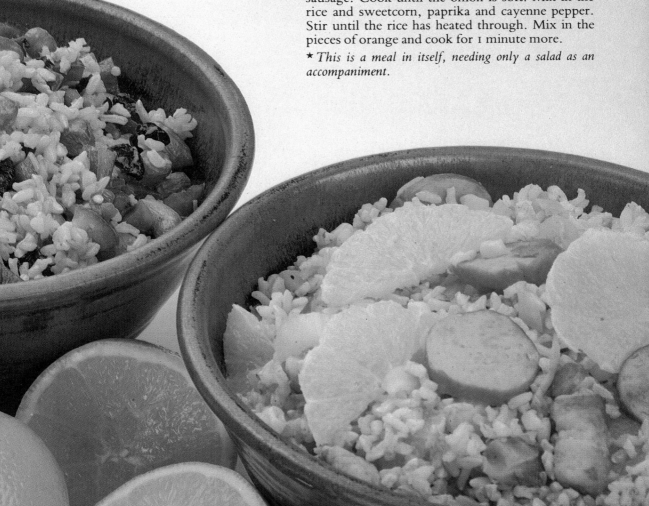

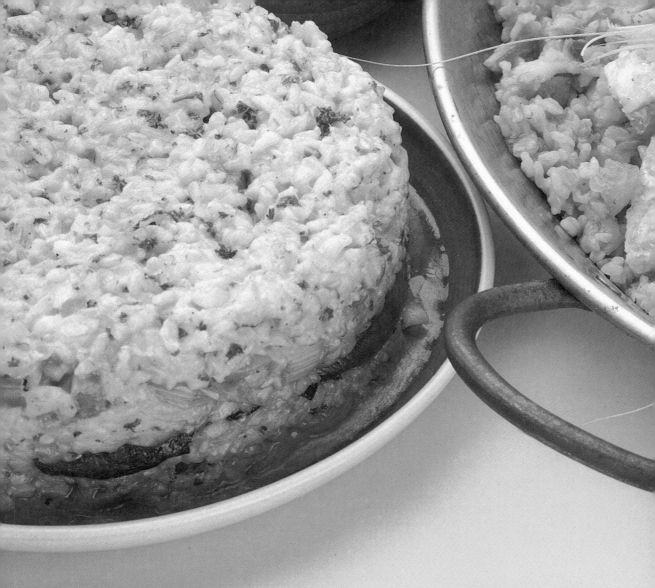

BROWN RICE AND MUSHROOM MOULD

225g/8 oz long grain brown rice
175g/6 oz grated Cheddar cheese
4 tbsp chopped parsley
freshly ground black pepper
225g/8 oz large flat mushrooms
40g/1½ oz butter and a little extra for greasing
4 large celery sticks, finely chopped
1 large onion, thinly sliced
1 garlic clove, finely chopped

Heat the oven to 110°C/225°F/Gas ¼. Cook the rice in lightly salted boiling water for about 45 minutes, or until tender. Drain but do not rinse the rice. While the rice is still hot, immediately fork in the cheese, parsley and pepper.

Remove the stalks from the mushrooms. Melt 25g/1 oz butter in a frying pan. Put in the mushrooms, fry quickly on both sides and remove. Melt the extra butter in the pan if necessary. Add the celery, onion and garlic and cook until the onion is soft.

Butter a 20-cm/8-in diameter soufflé dish. Put in a quarter of the rice in an even layer, then half the celery and onion, another quarter of the rice, all the mushrooms, the third quarter of the rice, the remaining celery and, finally, the remaining rice. Press down well. Bake the mould for 20 minutes.

To turn out, put a flat plate over the top of the dish. Turn the dish over and carefully lift it away.

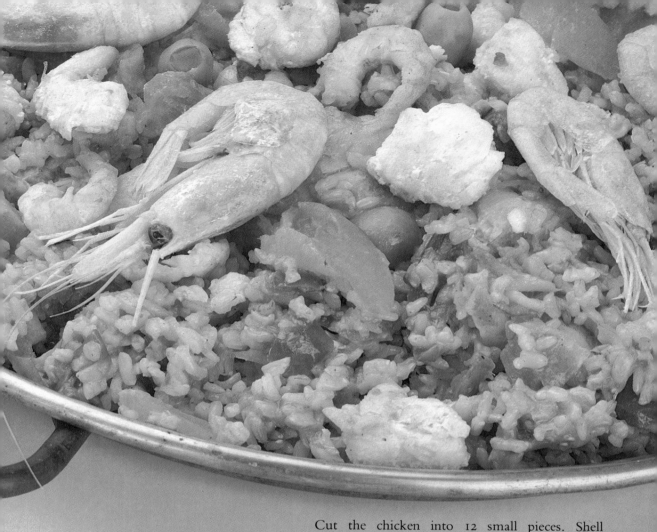

PARTY PAELLA

one 1.575-kg/3½-lb roasting chicken
675g/1½ lb prawns in shells
225g/8 oz cooked lean ham
450g/1 lb cod fillet
100ml/3½ fl oz olive oil
2 medium onions, finely chopped
1 garlic clove, finely chopped
2 red peppers, cored, seeded and cut into strips
2 green peppers, cored, seeded and cut into strips
2 tsp paprika
450g/1 lb long grain brown rice
¼ tsp saffron, soaked in 2 tbsp boiling water
1 litre/1¾ pints chicken stock
20 stuffed olives
350g/12 oz tomatoes, scalded, skinned, seeded and cut into strips
4 tbsp sherry
2 lemons, cut into wedges

Cut the chicken into 12 small pieces. Shell 450g/1 lb of the prawns. Finely dice the ham. Cut the cod into 2.5cm/1in pieces.

Heat the oil in a paella pan on a medium heat. Put in the cubes of cod, brown and remove. Add the onions, garlic, peppers and chicken pieces. Sprinkle in the paprika and cook for 10 minutes, stirring frequently.

Lower the heat. Add the rice and cook gently, stirring for 2 minutes. Add the saffron and water. Pour in the stock and bring to the boil. Add the ham. Cover the pan with a lid or foil and cook gently for 45 minutes, or until the rice is tender and all the stock absorbed.

Add the shelled prawns and the cod. Cover and cook for a further 10 minutes. Add the olives and tomatoes. Sprinkle in the sherry. Cook for a few minutes, uncovered, until the sherry has been absorbed.

Serve the paella straight from the pan, garnished with lemon wedges and the unshelled prawns.

★ *This paella will serve 10 people.*

MIXED BURGHUL SALAD

100g/4 oz burghul wheat
75g/3 oz watercress
1 large carrot
2 celery sticks
1 dessert apple
1 tsp tahini
2 tbsp oil
juice of ½ lemon
1 garlic clove, crushed with a pinch of sea salt
freshly ground black pepper

Soak the wheat in warm water for 20 minutes. Drain and squeeze dry. Chop the watercress, grate the carrot, chop the celery and core and chop the apple. Mix them into the wheat.

Beat the remaining ingredients together to make the dressing and fold into the salad.

★ *Tahini is a paste made from ground sesame seeds. It is available from most wholefood shops.*

BURGHUL, PEPPER AND MUSHROOM SALAD

225g/8 oz burghul wheat
1 red pepper
1 green pepper
100g/4 oz button mushrooms
4 tbsp olive oil
2 tbsp white wine vinegar
1 garlic clove, crushed with a pinch of sea salt
freshly ground black pepper

Soak the wheat in warm water for 20 minutes. Drain and squeeze dry. Core and seed the peppers and cut into strips. Thinly slice the mushrooms. Mix them into the wheat.

Beat the remaining ingredients together to make the dressing and fold into the salad. Leave the salad for 15 minutes before serving.

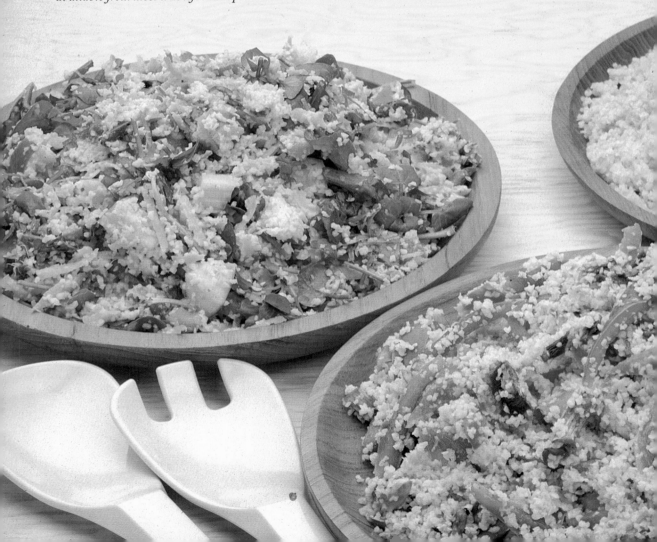

HOT BURGHUL

225g/8 oz burghul wheat
4 tbsp oil
1 medium onion, finely chopped
600ml/1 pint stock
sea salt
freshly ground black pepper

Heat the oil in a saucepan on a moderate heat. Stir in the burghul wheat and onion and cook for 2 minutes or until the burghul begins to brown.

Pour in the stock and bring to the boil. Season, cover and cook the burghul on a low heat for 10 minutes, so all the stock has been absorbed.

Turn off the heat and let the burghul stand for 10 minutes more.

★ *The final 10-minute standing period is not absolutely essential, but it gives the burghul a lighter fluffier texture.*

KASHA WITH MUSHROOMS

225g/8 oz buckwheat
3 tbsp oil
100g/4 oz mushrooms, finely chopped
1 large onion, thinly sliced
600ml/1 pint boiling water
½ tsp sea salt

Heat the oil in a frying pan on a low heat. Stir in the buckwheat, mushrooms and onion and cook, stirring frequently, until the buckwheat is a good brown. Pour in the water and bring to the boil. Add the salt.

Cover and set on a very low heat for 30 minutes.

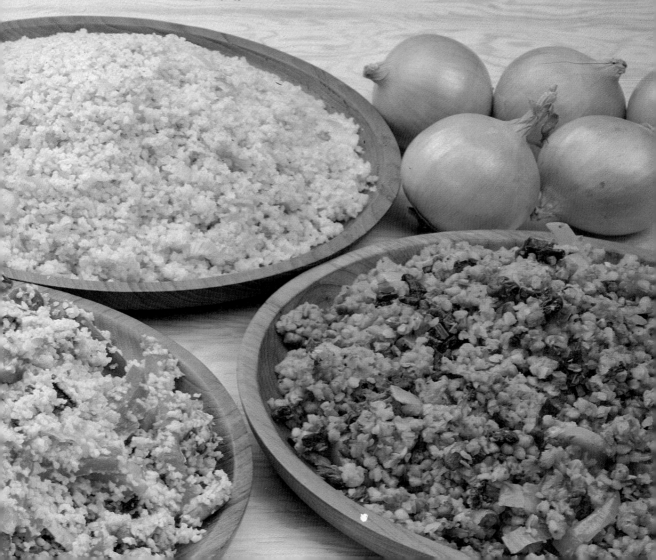

SPAGHETTI IN YOGHURT AND TOMATO SAUCE

225g/8 oz wholewheat spaghetti
4 tbsp natural yoghurt
1 tbsp tomato purée
1 garlic clove, crushed with a pinch of sea salt
freshly ground black pepper
1 tbsp chopped thyme

Cook the spaghetti in lightly salted boiling water for about 15 minutes, until it is just tender. While the spaghetti is cooking, mix together the yoghurt, tomato purée, garlic and pepper.

Drain the spaghetti, rinse with cold water and drain again. Return the spaghetti to the saucepan and gently mix in the yoghurt dressing and thyme.

Reheat, if necessary, on a very low heat, without boiling.

★ *Serve as an accompaniment to a main dish.*

WALNUT, SPAGHETTI AND AUBERGINES

675g/1½ lb aubergines
1 tbsp sea salt
450g/1 lb tomatoes
6 tbsp olive oil
1 large onion, quartered and thinly sliced
1 garlic clove, finely chopped
225g/8 oz wholewheat spaghetti
150g/5 oz walnuts
1 garlic clove, crushed with a pinch of sea salt
freshly ground black pepper
4 tbsp chopped parsley
100g/4 oz grated Cheddar cheese (optional)

Cut the aubergines into 1cm/½in dice. Put the aubergines into a colander, scatter with the salt and leave to drain for 20 minutes. Rinse with cold water and dry with kitchen paper. Scald, skin and chop the tomatoes.

Heat 3 tbsp oil in a saucepan on a low heat. Put in the onion and chopped garlic and cook until they begin to look transparent. Stir in the aubergines, cover and cook for 5 minutes. Add the tomatoes, cover again and cook for 10 minutes. Keep warm.

While the vegetables are cooking, boil the spaghetti in lightly salted water until it is tender. Drain, rinse with cold water and drain again. Coarsely crush or finely chop the walnuts.

Melt the remaining oil in a saucepan on a low heat. Stir in the crushed garlic and cook until it begins to sizzle. Gently fold in the spaghetti and reheat. Add the parsley and season well with pepper.

Divide the spaghetti between 4 individual plates and spoon over the aubergines and tomatoes. Scatter the grated cheese on top, if using.

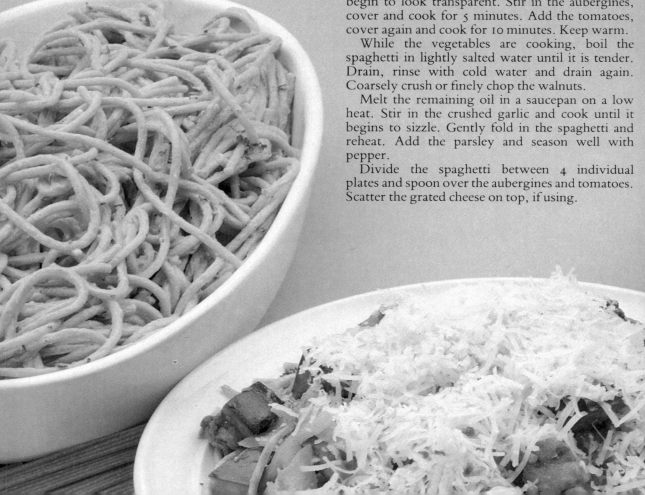

SARDINE SPAGHETTI

275g/10 oz wholewheat spaghetti
four 120-g/4¼-oz tins sardines in oil
450g/1 lb tomatoes
16 black olives
2 tbsp olive oil
1 large onion, quartered and thinly sliced
1 garlic clove, finely chopped
2 tbsp grated Parmesan cheese
2 tbsp chopped parsley

Cook the spaghetti in lightly salted boiling water for about 15 minutes, or until tender. Drain, rinse with hot water and drain again.

While the spaghetti is cooking, drain and flake the sardines, scald, skin and chop the tomatoes, and halve and stone the olives. Heat the oil in a saucepan on a low heat. Put in the onion and garlic and cook until they are just beginning to brown. Fold in the spaghetti, sardines, tomatoes and olives and heat through.

Turn the spaghetti out either into 1 large serving dish or onto 4 individual plates. Scatter the Parmesan cheese and parsley over the top.

TAGLIATELLE WITH SALAMI AND CHEESE

275g/10 oz wholewheat tagliatelle
225g/8 oz peppercorn-coated salami, thinly sliced
4 tbsp olive oil
1 large onion, quartered and thinly sliced
1 garlic clove, finely chopped
350g/12 oz tomatoes, scalded, skinned and chopped
2 tbsp grated Parmesan cheese
4 tbsp chopped parsley
175g/6 oz grated Gruyère cheese

Cook the tagliatelle in lightly salted boiling water for about 12 minutes, or until tender. Drain, rinse with hot water, drain again and keep warm.

Chop the salami. Heat the oil in a saucepan on a low heat. Put in the onion, garlic and salami and cook until the onion is soft. Mix in the tagliatelle, tomatoes, Parmesan cheese and parsley and cook for 1 minute so the tomatoes just heat through.

Heat the grill to high. Turn the mixture onto a heatproof serving dish and scatter the Gruyère cheese over the top. Put the dish under the grill for the cheese to melt.

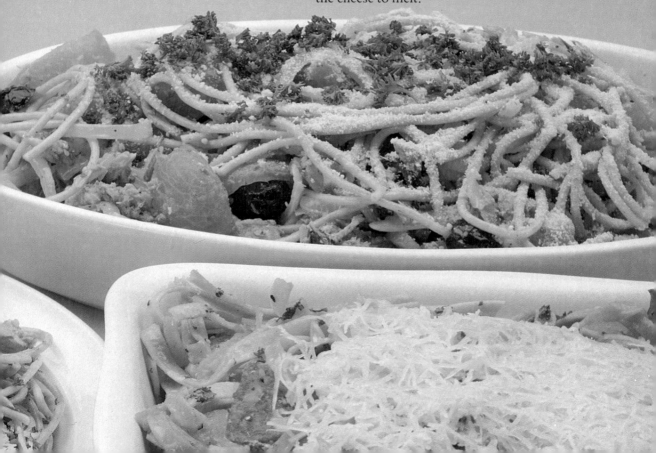

SAVOURY WHEAT CASSEROLE

225g/8 oz wheat grains
25g/1 oz butter
1 large onion, finely chopped
4 celery sticks, finely chopped
100g/4 oz flat mushrooms, thinly sliced
200ml/7 fl oz stock
2 tbsp Worcestershire sauce
4 tbsp chopped parsley
75g/3 oz Red Leicester cheese, finely grated

Boil the wheat grains in salted water for 1 hour. Drain.

Heat the oven to 200°C/400°F/Gas 6. Melt the butter in a casserole on a low heat. Mix in the onion and celery and cook until the onion is soft. Mix in the wheat and mushrooms and pour in the stock. Add the Worcestershire sauce and fork in the parsley and cheese. Cover the casserole and put it into the oven for 30 minutes.

★ *To make the dish into a main course: use 225g/8oz cheese. Fork 75g/3oz cheese into the casserole. After 20 minutes of cooking remove the lid and scatter the remaining cheese over the top of the wheat. Cook for a further 10 minutes, uncovered.*

BARLEY AND CARROT BAKE

225g/8 oz pot barley
350g/12 oz carrots
4 tomatoes
2 large onions
4 tbsp sunflower oil
½ tsp cayenne pepper
600ml/1 pint stock
½ tsp sea salt
2 tbsp chopped thyme
2 tbsp chopped parsley

Heat the oven to 200°C/400°F/Gas 6. Finely dice the carrots. Scald, skin and chop the tomatoes and finely chop the onions.

Heat the oil in a flameproof casserole on a low heat. Mix in the onions and carrots and cook until the onions are soft. Mix in the tomatoes, barley and cayenne pepper and stir for 1 minute. Pour in the stock and bring to the boil. Season with the salt and stir in the herbs.

Cover the casserole and cook in the oven for 45 minutes so all the stock is absorbed and the barley is soft.

★ *Serve as an accompaniment to a main dish.*

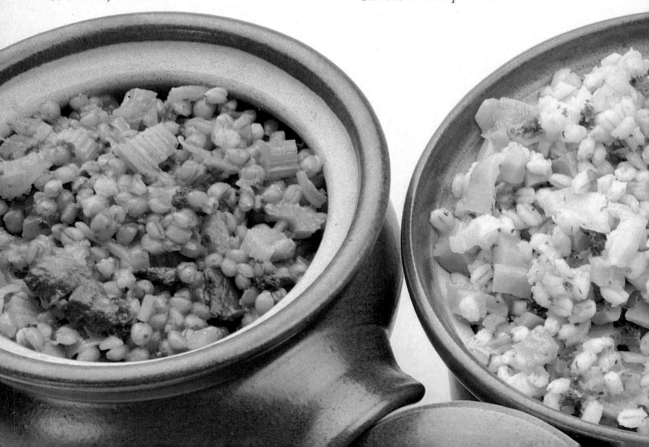

BARLEY BROTH WITH LEEKS

900-g/2-lb neck of lamb, chopped into small pieces

BOILING
1.5 litres/2½ pints water
1 small onion, halved
1 small carrot, roughly chopped
bouquet garni
2 bayleaves
2 tsp black peppercorns

SOUP
50g/2 oz pot barley
175g/6 oz carrots
350g/12 oz leeks
4 tbsp chopped parsley

Put the lamb into a large saucepan with the boiling ingredients. Set on a moderate heat, bring to the boil and skim. Cover and simmer for 1 hour 30 minutes. Strain and reserve the stock. Reserve the lamb and discard the onion, carrot and herbs.

Put the stock into a clean saucepan and bring to the boil. Put in the barley, cover and simmer for 30 minutes. Remove the lamb from the bones and chop finely. Finely chop the carrots and thinly slice the leeks. Put the carrots and meat into the saucepan and simmer for a further 30 minutes. Add the leeks and parsley and cook 10 minutes more.

Serve in large bowls as a main meal.

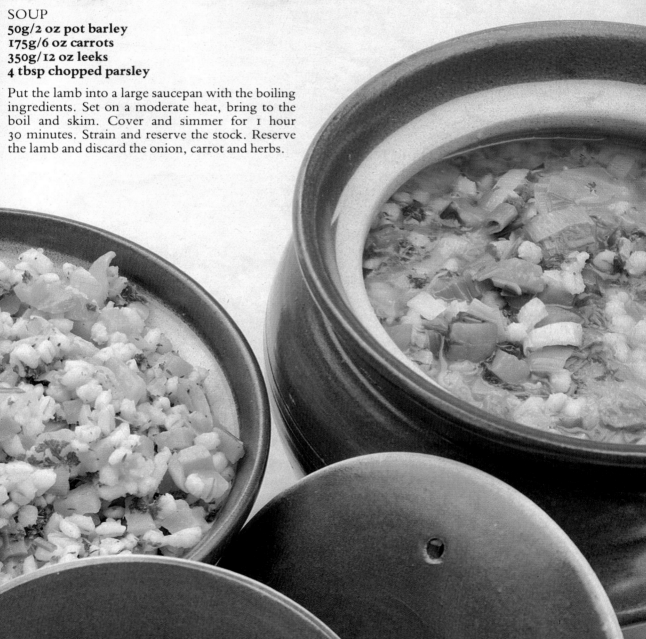

SALADS AND VEGETABLES

All vegetables contain fibre so several kinds should be included in every meal. They can be served either as an accompaniment to or as the base for the main dish. The nearer vegetables are to their natural state, the more fibre they contain, so buy them fresh rather than tinned or frozen. When preparing vegetables, only peel them when absolutely necessary, get them ready just before starting to cook or to make a salad and do not leave them soaking in water for long periods.

Use sharp knives to shred or slice vegetables to make fresh, crispy salads. Mix several types together and add chopped fresh fruits, small dried fruits and chopped nuts for extra variety. Different kinds of oils and vinegars can be mixed to make the dressings, and you can also add small amounts of sauces, tomato purée or spices.

Vegetables should never be overcooked. Boil them in the minimum amount of water, or lightly steam them, and in both cases only cook vegetables until they are just tender. Simmering in butter or oil are other good, quick ways of cooking vegetables and they can also be stir-fried or baked in parcels of foil.

Always cook potatoes with their skins on and when they are baked in their jackets, eat the skins as well.

CHICORY, TOMATO AND WALNUT SALAD

3 heads chicory
450g/1 lb tomatoes
50g/2 oz shelled walnuts
4 tbsp oil
2 tbsp white wine vinegar
1 garlic clove, crushed with a pinch of sea salt
freshly ground black pepper
2 tbsp chopped parsley

Cut the chicory heads in half and thinly slice each half. Put the slices in the centre of a serving plate. Thinly slice the tomatoes and arrange them round the edge.

Finely chop the walnuts and scatter over the chicory only. Beat together the oil, vinegar, garlic and pepper and spoon the dressing over the salad. Scatter the parsley over the tomatoes.

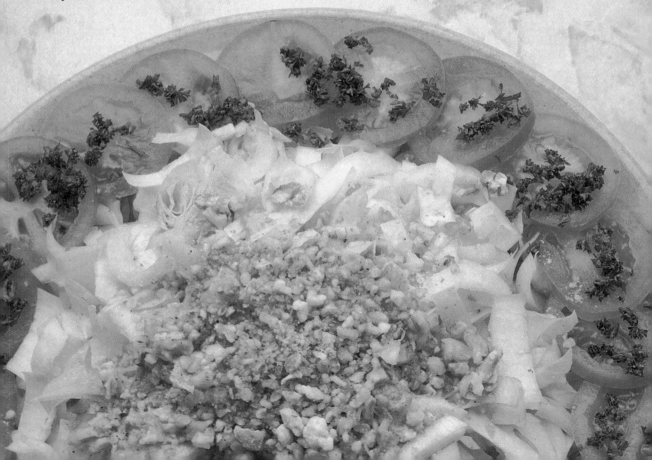

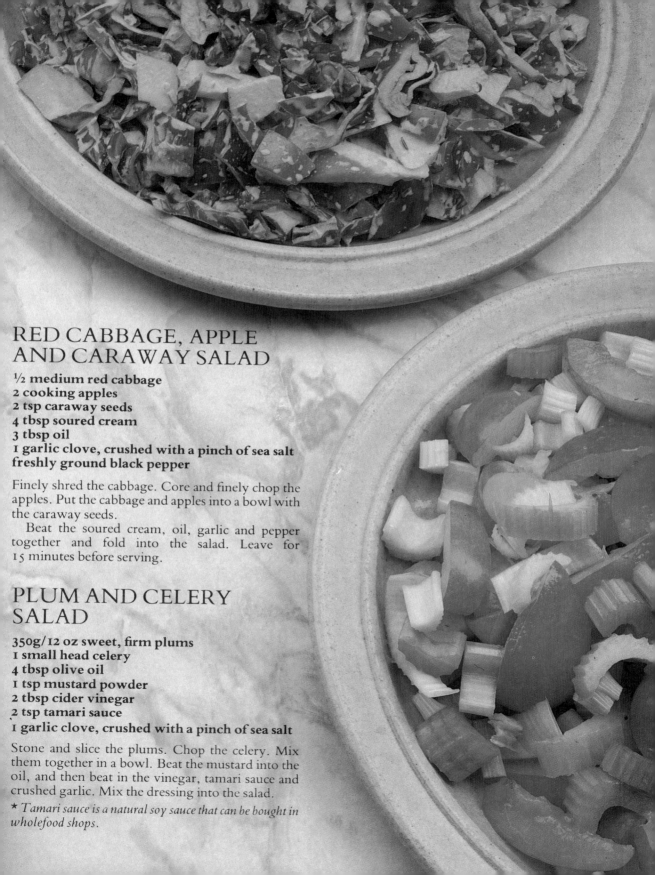

RED CABBAGE, APPLE
AND CARAWAY SALAD

½ medium red cabbage
2 cooking apples
2 tsp caraway seeds
4 tbsp soured cream
3 tbsp oil
I garlic clove, crushed with a pinch of sea salt
freshly ground black pepper

Finely shred the cabbage. Core and finely chop the
apples. Put the cabbage and apples into a bowl with
the caraway seeds.

   Beat the soured cream, oil, garlic and pepper
together and fold into the salad. Leave for
15 minutes before serving.

PLUM AND CELERY
SALAD

350g/12 oz sweet, firm plums
I small head celery
4 tbsp olive oil
I tsp mustard powder
2 tbsp cider vinegar
2 tsp tamari sauce
I garlic clove, crushed with a pinch of sea salt

Stone and slice the plums. Chop the celery. Mix
them together in a bowl. Beat the mustard into the
oil, and then beat in the vinegar, tamari sauce and
crushed garlic. Mix the dressing into the salad.

★ *Tamari sauce is a natural soy sauce that can be bought in
wholefood shops.*

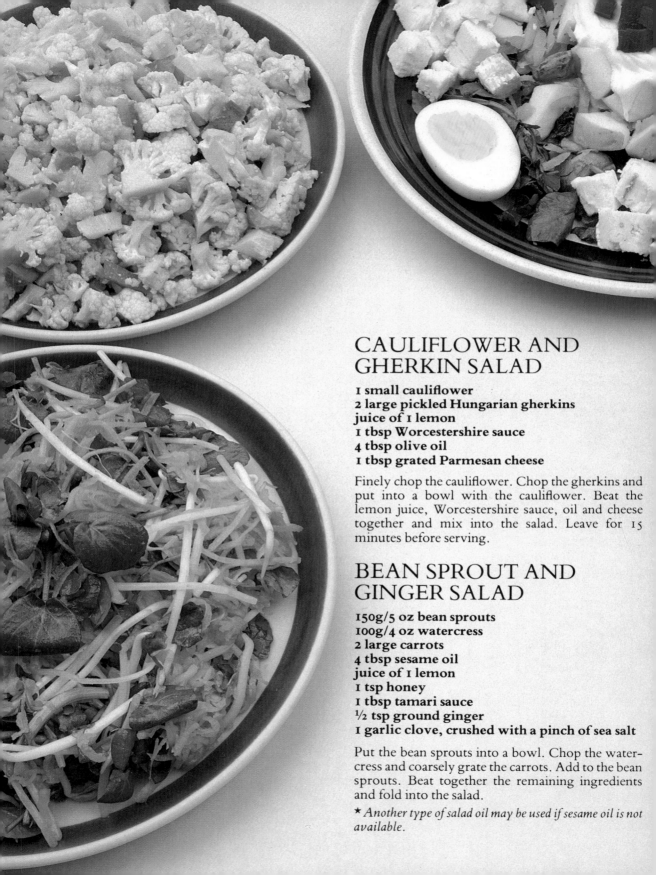

CAULIFLOWER AND GHERKIN SALAD

1 small cauliflower
2 large pickled Hungarian gherkins
juice of 1 lemon
1 tbsp Worcestershire sauce
4 tbsp olive oil
1 tbsp grated Parmesan cheese

Finely chop the cauliflower. Chop the gherkins and put into a bowl with the cauliflower. Beat the lemon juice, Worcestershire sauce, oil and cheese together and mix into the salad. Leave for 15 minutes before serving.

BEAN SPROUT AND GINGER SALAD

150g/5 oz bean sprouts
100g/4 oz watercress
2 large carrots
4 tbsp sesame oil
juice of 1 lemon
1 tsp honey
1 tbsp tamari sauce
½ tsp ground ginger
1 garlic clove, crushed with a pinch of sea salt

Put the bean sprouts into a bowl. Chop the watercress and coarsely grate the carrots. Add to the bean sprouts. Beat together the remaining ingredients and fold into the salad.

★ *Another type of salad oil may be used if sesame oil is not available.*

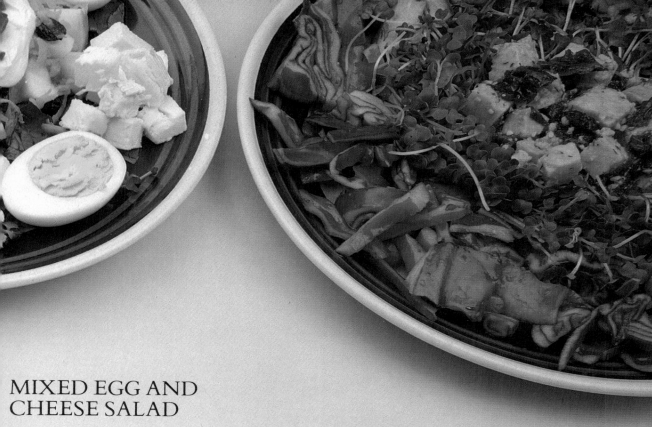

MIXED EGG AND CHEESE SALAD

8 eggs
150g/5 oz soft cheese such as Brie or
    Camembert
150g/5 oz soft blue cheese such as Lymeswold
    or blue Brie
2 bunches watercress
225g/8 oz carrots
1 cooking apple
50g/2 oz peanuts
50g/2 oz raisins
50g/2 oz curd cheese
4 tbsp mayonnaise
6 tbsp natural yoghurt
¼ tsp mustard powder
175g/6 oz beetroot, cooked

Hard boil the eggs and halve them lengthways.
Dice the cheeses. Chop the watercress and divide
between 4 plates, putting it in the centre. Grate
the carrots and core and chop the apple. Mix with
the peanuts and raisins and put on top of the watercress.

    Beat together the curd cheese, mayonnaise,
yoghurt and mustard powder. Spoon the dressing
over the carrot salad.

    Arrange diced white cheese on one side of the
salad and blue cheese on the other. Put the eggs in
between the cheeses. Finely dice the beetroot and
use as a garnish on top of the salad.

RED WINDSOR AND PRUNE SALAD

6 prunes
6 tbsp dry red wine
2 tbsp chopped thyme
1 garlic clove, crushed with a pinch of sea salt
1 tbsp red wine vinegar
4 tbsp oil
½ medium red cabbage
175g/6 oz Red Windsor cheese
50g/2 oz alfalfa sprouts or 2 boxes of salad cress

Soak the prunes in the wine for at least 6 hours.
Stone and chop the prunes. Beat the thyme, garlic,
wine vinegar and oil into the wine.

    Finely shred the cabbage and put into a bowl.
Mix in half the dressing and leave to stand for
30 minutes.

    Cut the cheese into 1cm/½in dice. Arrange the
cabbage in a ring on 4 fairly large serving plates and
put a bed of alfalfa or cress in the centre.

    Mix the prunes and cheese into the remaining
dressing and arrange them on top of the alfalfa or
cress.

★ *Serve as a light lunch or supper dish.*

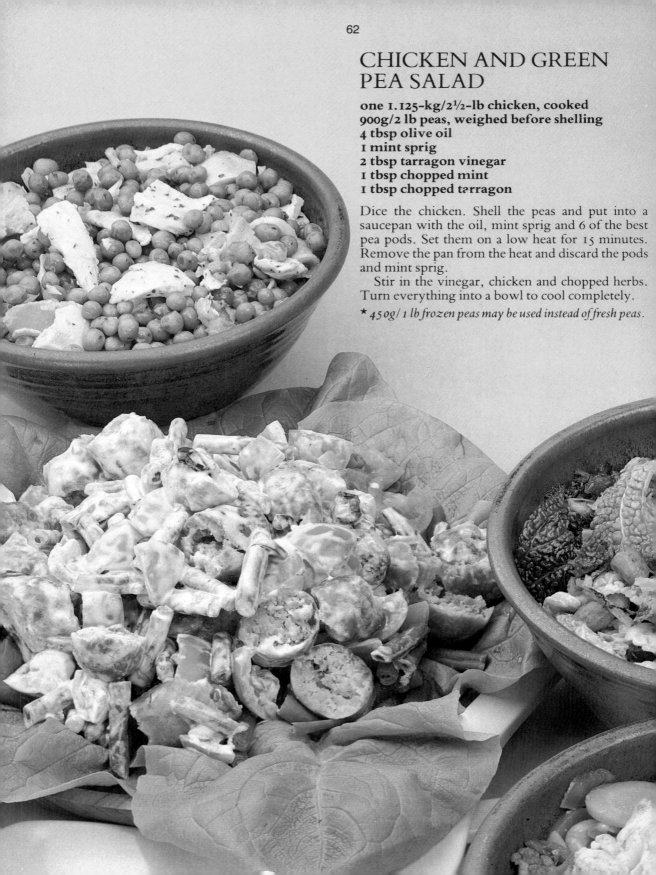

CHICKEN AND GREEN PEA SALAD

one 1.125-kg/2½-lb chicken, cooked
900g/2 lb peas, weighed before shelling
4 tbsp olive oil
1 mint sprig
2 tbsp tarragon vinegar
1 tbsp chopped mint
1 tbsp chopped tarragon

Dice the chicken. Shell the peas and put into a saucepan with the oil, mint sprig and 6 of the best pea pods. Set them on a low heat for 15 minutes. Remove the pan from the heat and discard the pods and mint sprig.

Stir in the vinegar, chicken and chopped herbs. Turn everything into a bowl to cool completely.

★ *450g/1 lb frozen peas may be used instead of fresh peas.*

FRENCH BEAN AND SAUSAGE SALAD

675g/1½ lb 100% pork sausages
450g/1 lb French beans
2 tsp chopped thyme
450g/1 lb tomatoes
10 black olives
2 tbsp natural yoghurt
2 tbsp mayonnaise
1 lettuce

Grill the sausages until brown and cooked through. Cool. Top and tail the beans. Put the beans into a saucepan with the thyme and 2cm/¾in water. Cover and set on a moderate heat for 20 minutes, turning occasionally. Drain and cool.

Chop the tomatoes. Stone and quarter the olives. Cut the beans into 2-cm/¾-in lengths and the sausages into thin slices. Combine the sausages, beans, tomatoes and olives in a bowl.

Mix together the yoghurt and mayonnaise. Mix into the salad. Arrange the lettuce on a large serving dish and pile the salad on top.

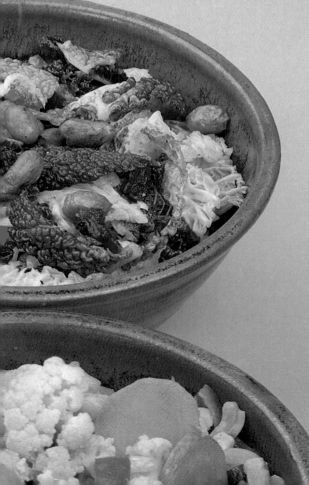

STIR-FRIED SAVOY WITH PEANUTS AND DATES

1 medium Savoy cabbage
4 tbsp oil
1 garlic clove, finely chopped
175g–225g/6 oz–8 oz peanuts
75g/3 oz stoned dried dates, chopped
2 tbsp white wine vinegar
2 tsp Dijon mustard

Finely shred the cabbage. Heat the oil and garlic in a wok or a large frying pan on a high heat until the garlic begins to sizzle.

Mix in the cabbage, peanuts and dates and stir fry for about 2 minutes until the cabbage is wilted and is a bright, fresh green. Stir in the vinegar and mustard and keep stirring for another minute, lowering the heat if the cabbage shows any sign of browning.

Take the pan from the heat. Serve as soon as possible, as a main course.

STIR-BRAISED VEGETABLES WITH CASHEW NUTS

1 medium cauliflower
175g/6 oz carrots
1 small green pepper
1 small red pepper
1 large onion
3 tbsp dry sherry
2 tbsp tamari sauce
1 tbsp white wine vinegar
1 tbsp tomato purée
1 tsp honey
4 tbsp oil
1 garlic clove, finely chopped
175g–225g/6 oz–8 oz cashew nuts

Cut the cauliflower into very small florets. Thinly slice the carrots. Core and seed the peppers and cut into 2.5cm/1in strips. Finely chop the onion. Mix together the sherry, tamari, vinegar, tomato purée and honey.

Heat the oil and garlic in a wok or large frying pan until the garlic begins to sizzle. Mix in the vegetables and stir fry for 2 minutes. Mix in the cashew nuts and stir fry for another minute. Pour in the sherry mixture and bring to the boil. Cover and keep on a moderate heat for 10 minutes. Serve as soon as possible.

★ Tamari sauce is a natural soy sauce that can be bought in wholefood shops.

BAKED POTATOES WITH PARSLEY AND ONION

4 baking potatoes
50g/2 oz butter
4 tbsp chopped parsley
sea salt
freshly ground black pepper
1 large onion, finely chopped

Heat the oven to 200°C/400°F/Gas 6. Scrub the potatoes and prick with a fork. Lay them on the oven rack and bake for 1 hour 30 minutes or until the skins are crisp.

Cut each potato in half lengthways. Scoop out the middles and mash with the butter. Mix in the parsley and season.

Pile the mixture back into the potato shells and scatter the chopped onion over the top. Return the potatoes to the oven for 15 minutes to brown.

BRUSSELS SPROUTS WITH DIJON MUSTARD

450g/1 lb Brussels sprouts
1 tbsp Dijon mustard
2 tbsp chopped parsley

Trim the sprouts and simmer in lightly salted water for 10 minutes. Drain and return to the saucepan. Set on a low heat and stir in the mustard and parsley.

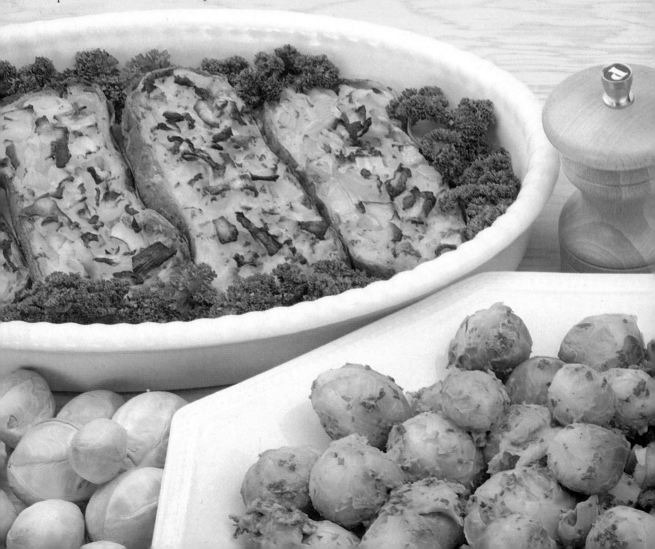

SPRING GREENS, LEEKS AND ROSEMARY

225g/8 oz spring greens
225g/8 oz leeks
15g/½ oz butter
2 tsp chopped rosemary
150ml/¼ pint water

Chop the spring greens and thinly slice the leeks. Melt the butter in a saucepan on a high heat. Mix in the vegetables and rosemary. Pour in the water and bring to the boil. Cover and cook on a low heat for 20 minutes.

CARROTS IN A PACKET

450g/1 lb carrots
1 medium onion
butter for greasing
grated rind of 1 small orange
1 tbsp chopped thyme
sea salt
freshly ground black pepper

Heat the oven to 180°C/350°F/Gas 4. Finely chop the carrots and onion. Lay the vegetables in the centre of a piece of buttered aluminium foil approximately 37.5cm/15in square. Sprinkle on the orange rind. Scatter the thyme on top and season. Bring the sides of the foil together and fold to seal them. Fold over the ends.

Lay the foil parcel on a baking sheet and bake in the oven for 1 hour 15 minutes. Tip the carrots into a warmed dish to serve.

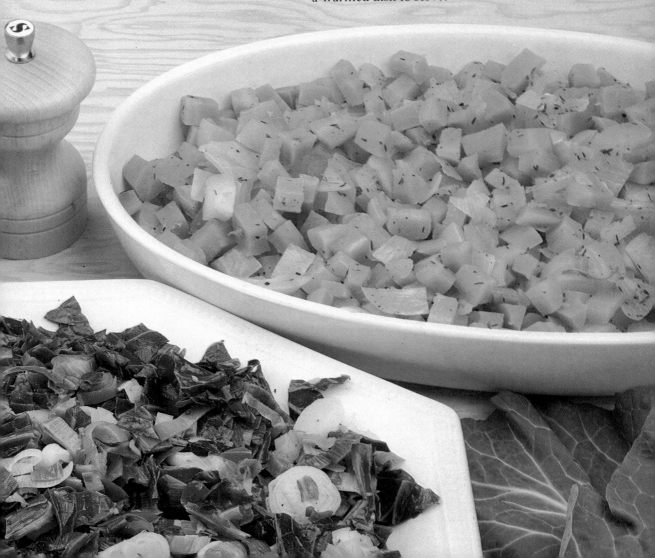

DESERTS

High-fibre desserts need not be heavy if you base them on fresh and dried fruits, both of which are good sources of fibre.

Use fresh and dried fruit separately or mix them together to make fruit salads or cook gently to make compotes. Grill or bake fruit or use it to make more elaborate dishes such as fruit fools and sylla-bubs. When making fruit pies, flans or cobbler dishes, use wholewheat flour. Use granary or wholewheat bread to make a version of summer pudding and use a muesli base to make a crumble topping or flan base.

Short grain brown rice, flaked brown rice or wholewheat semolina can be used in the same way as the white types to make milk puddings.

RHUBARB CRUMBLE

450g/1 lb rhubarb
50g/2 oz sultanas
50g/2 oz demerara sugar
75g/3 oz muesli base (p.6)
15g/½ oz wheatgerm
15g/½ oz chopped toasted hazelnuts
25g/1 oz desiccated coconut
3 tbsp sunflower oil

Heat the oven to 200°C/400°F/Gas 6. Finely chop the rhubarb and mix with the sultanas and sugar. Put them into a pie dish.

Mix together the remaining ingredients, making sure the oil coats the rest well. Put on top of the rhubarb mixture so it is covered completely.

Bake the crumble for 30 minutes so the top is golden brown. Serve it hot or cold.

DRIED FRUIT AND PINEAPPLE SALAD

100g/4 oz dried apricots
100g/4 oz dried prunes
300ml/½ pint natural pineapple juice
1 medium pineapple

Soak the apricots and prunes in the pineapple juice for at least 8 hours. Halve and stone the prunes and return to the liquid.

Cut the husk from the pineapple. Cut the flesh into 1cm/½in slices and stamp out the cores. Cut the slices into 2.5cm/1in pieces and mix into the dried fruits. Leave for 1 hour before serving.

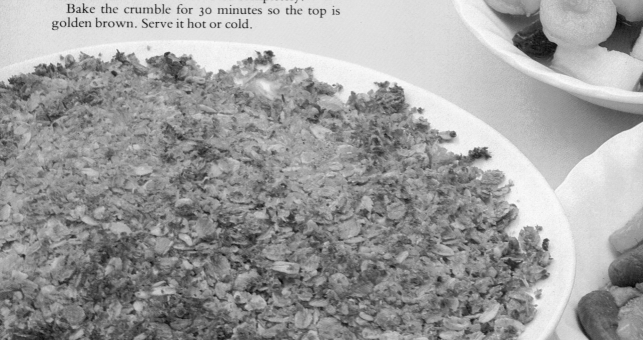

FIGS AND ORANGES IN RED WINE

12 dried figs
300ml/½ pint dry red wine
2 tbsp honey
2 large oranges

Put the wine, honey and a thinly pared strip of orange rind into a saucepan. Stir on a low heat until the honey has melted. Bring to simmering point and add the figs. Cover and cook very gently for 15 minutes. Cool.

Cut the rind and pith from the oranges. Cut each orange in half lengthways and thinly slice the halves. Add the oranges to the figs. Chill for 30 minutes before serving.

BLACKBERRY PUDDING

1 large loaf granary bread, 2 days old
350g/12 oz blackberries
3 tbsp honey
5cm/2in cinnamon stick
150ml/¼ pint natural yoghurt
or soured cream

Cut the bread into thin slices. Use the slices to line a 600ml/1 pint pudding basin, saving enough to cover the top. Put the blackberries, honey and cinnamon stick into a saucepan and set on a very low heat for about 5 minutes, so the juices begin to run from the blackberries and the honey is melted. Remove the cinnamon stick. Tip all the blackberries and their juice into the lined basin. Cover the top with the reserved bread.

Put a flat plate over the basin and weight it down. Leave the pudding for 12 hours.

Chill the pudding for 30 minutes. Turn it out. Serve the yoghurt or soured cream separately.

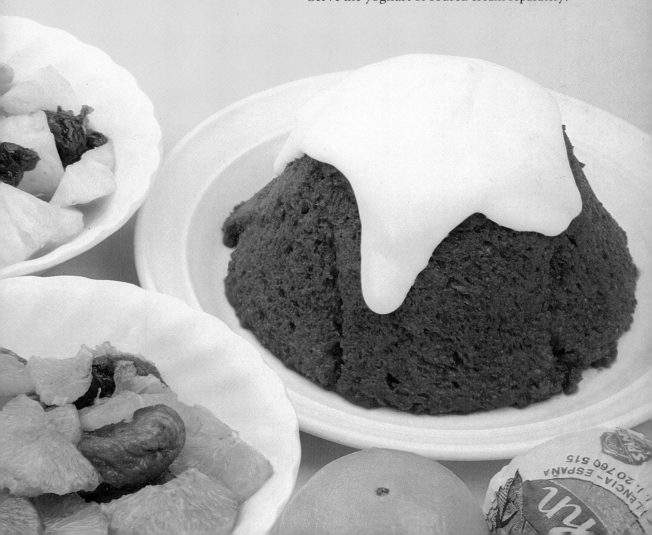

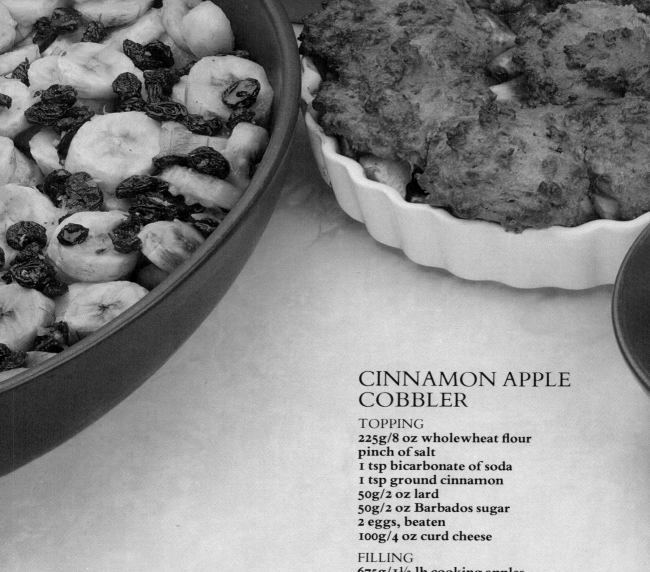

CINNAMON APPLE COBBLER

TOPPING
**225g/8 oz wholewheat flour
pinch of salt
1 tsp bicarbonate of soda
1 tsp ground cinnamon
50g/2 oz lard
50g/2 oz Barbados sugar
2 eggs, beaten
100g/4 oz curd cheese**

FILLING
**675g/1½ lb cooking apples
50g/2 oz Barbados sugar
1 tsp ground cinnamon**

Heat the oven to 190°C/375°F/Gas 5. Put the flour, salt, bicarbonate of soda and cinnamon into a bowl and rub in the lard. Toss in the sugar with your fingers and make a well in the centre. Add the eggs and curd cheese and, using a wooden spoon, beat everything to a smooth, moist dough.

Peel, core and chop the apples and mix in a bowl with the sugar and cinnamon. Put the filling into a 20cm/8in flan dish. Spoon the cobbler topping on top in portions of about 2 tbsp each, keeping them separate if possible. There should be 12–15 portions.

Bake the cobbler for 40 minutes, so the scones rise and turn golden brown. Serve hot with single cream or custard.

BANANAS BAKED IN SHERRY

**6 bananas
50g/2 oz raisins
grated rind and juice of 1 medium orange
6 tbsp sweet sherry
butter for greasing
yoghurt or soured cream for serving**

Heat the oven to 200°C/400°F/Gas 6. Slice the bananas into 6-mm/¼-in thick rounds. Put into a small pie dish and mix in the raisins and orange rind. Pour in the orange juice and sherry.

Cover the dish with lightly buttered foil and bake in the oven for 20 minutes. Serve the bananas hot, with yoghurt or soured cream served separately.

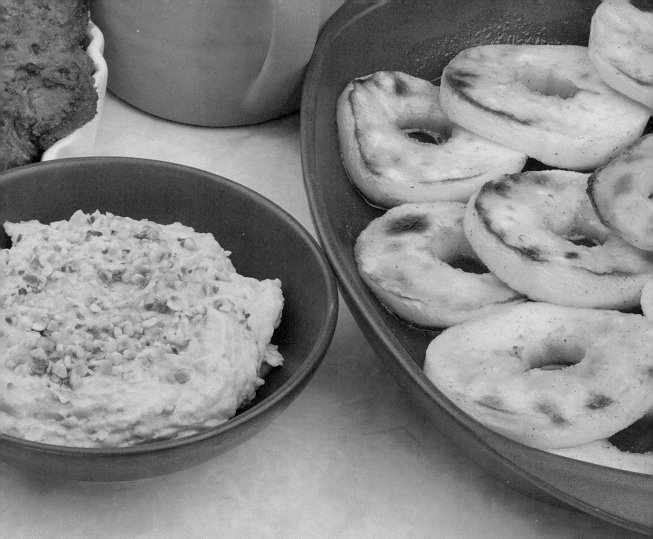

DRIED FRUIT SYLLABUB

150g/5 oz dried apricots
50g/2 oz prunes
300ml/½ pint natural orange juice
300ml/½ pint double cream
3 tbsp whisky
2 tbsp chopped toasted hazelnuts

Soak the apricots and prunes in the orange juice for at least 12 hours.

Stone the prunes. Put the apricots, prunes and orange juice into a blender and work to a purée. Whip the cream with the whisky until light and fluffy and fold into the fruit. Pile the mixture into individual dishes and scatter the toasted hazelnuts over the top.

★ *Some wholefood shops sell ready toasted chopped hazelnuts. If they are not available, put whole hazelnuts on a baking tray and cook in a 180°C/350°F/Gas 4 oven for 20 minutes. Cool and chop.*

GRILLED APPLE SLICES WITH SPICED HONEY

4 medium–large cooking apples
25g/1 oz butter, melted
3 tbsp honey
½ tsp ground mixed spice

Peel and core the apples. Cut into 6-mm/¼-in thick rings and lay on a flat, heatproof dish, overlapping as little as possible. Brush them with the melted butter. Put the honey into a saucepan with the spice and melt on a low heat. Spoon the honey over the apples.

Heat the grill to high. Put the dish under the grill so the apples are about 5cm/2in from the heat. Grill until the top is brown and bubbling, turn and grill the other side.

SNACKS AND SWEETS

Snack meals and between meals nibbles can all be made from high-fibre ingredients.

Many quick and easy meals can be based on wholewheat bread. Make it into single and double-decker sandwiches or toast it and put other high-fibre ingredients such as cooked beans on top. Rye breads made from whole rye flour can be used for delicious and attractive open sandwiches.

To satisfy a sweet tooth make chewy bars from muesli base or rolled oats, and mix dried fruits and nuts to make high-fibre confectionery.

LIVER SAUSAGE OPEN SANDWICHES

TO MAKE FOUR SANDWICHES
175g/6 oz liver sausage
25g/1 oz butter
4 slices rye bread
4 spring onions, finely chopped
4 stuffed olives
4 radish slices

In a bowl, cream together 50g/2 oz of liver sausage and the butter. Spread this mixture thickly over the slices of bread. Press the chopped spring onions on top. Cut the remaining liver sausage into 4 slices. Put a slice onto the centre of each slice of bread.

Cut each olive into 4 slices. Use these and the radish slices to garnish the liver sausage.

CORN SCRAMBLE ON TOAST

one 350-g/12-oz tin sweetcorn
50g/2 oz butter
1 large onion, quartered and thinly sliced
4 celery sticks, finely chopped
8 eggs, beaten
100g/4 oz grated Cheddar cheese
pinch of cayenne pepper
½ tsp paprika
8 large slices wholewheat bread, toasted and buttered

Drain the sweetcorn. Melt the butter in a saucepan on a low heat. Stir in the onion and celery and cook until soft. Stir in the eggs, cheese and sweetcorn and season with the pepper. Cook for about 3 minutes, stirring continuously, until the eggs set to a light scramble.

Pile the scramble onto the hot buttered toast and sprinkle with a little paprika.

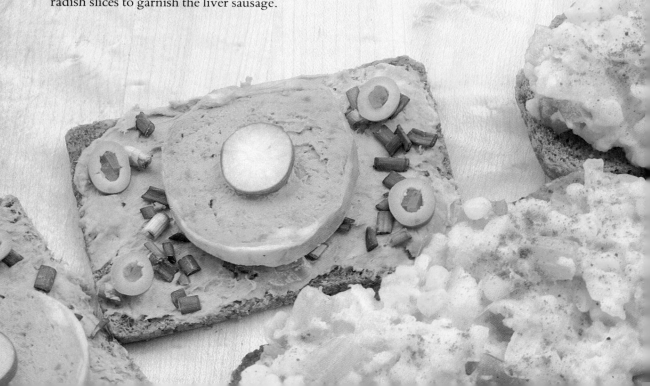

CORNED BEEF HASH

225g/8 oz corned beef, sliced
575g/1¼ lb potatoes
1 medium onion, thinly sliced
50g/2 oz butter
6 tbsp milk
2 tsp tomato purée
¼ tsp Tabasco sauce
pinch of sea salt
3 tbsp chopped parsley

Boil the potatoes in their skins with the onion. Drain and skin the potatoes. Mash with the onion, half the butter, the milk, tomato purée, Tabasco sauce and salt. Finely chop the corned beef and mix into the potato.

Melt the remaining butter in a large frying pan on a moderate heat. Put in the potato mixture and press down in an even layer. Cook until the underside browns. Turn the hash over in sections. Let the underside brown again. Mix the browned parts into the rest and repeat the browning twice more. Mix again and serve.

★ *A tomato salad is a good accompaniment.*

JACKET POTATOES WITH STILTON CHEESE

4 large potatoes
100g/4 oz grated Stilton cheese
1 egg, beaten
25g/1 oz butter
2 tbsp chopped parsley

Heat the oven to 200°C/400°F/Gas 6. Scrub the potatoes, prick on both sides and bake on the oven rack for 1 hour 30 minutes or until the middles are soft and the outsides crisp.

Cut the potatoes in half lengthways and scoop out the centres. Mash and mix in the cheese, egg, butter and parsley.

Pile the mixture back into the potato shells. Put the shells onto a heatproof serving dish and return to the oven for 10 minutes, for the tops to brown.

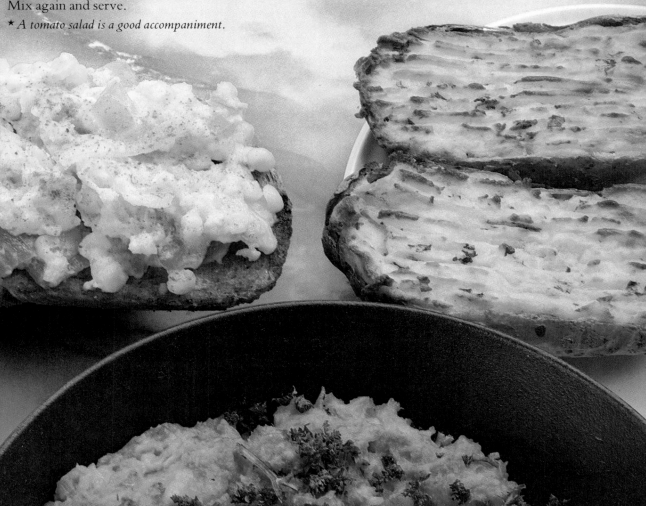

CHEWY HAZELNUT BARS

100g/4 oz shelled hazelnuts, finely chopped
225g/8 oz muesli base
75g/3 oz sultanas
100g/4 oz light Barbados sugar
2 tbsp honey
125ml/4 fl oz sunflower oil
  plus extra for greasing

Heat the oven to 200°C/400°F/Gas 6. Mix together the hazelnuts, muesli base and sultanas. Put the sugar, honey and oil into a saucepan and set on a low heat. Stir until the honey and sugar have melted and the oil is well incorporated. Add the hazelnuts, muesli and sultanas and mix well.

Press the mixture into a well-oiled 20 × 28cm/ 8 × 11in baking tin. Put into the oven for 10 minutes.

Cut the mixture into bars and leave in the tin until the bars are just warm so they set into shape. Remove to a wire rack or a flat plate and leave until they are completely cold.

BRAZIL NUT SWEETS

100g/4 oz shelled Brazil nuts
100g/4 oz dessert figs
100g/4 oz stoned dates
rice paper

Finely mince together the Brazil nuts, figs and dates. Work the mixture well with your fingers to ensure the ingredients are evenly mixed.

Roll out the mixture between sheets of rice paper to a thickness of 6mm/¼in. Cut into 2.5cm/1in squares or small bars.

APRICOT SWEETS

225g/8 oz dried apricots
150ml/¼ pint unsweetened orange juice
75g/3 oz raisins
100g/4 oz sunflower seeds
rice paper

Soak the apricots in the orange juice for 2 hours. Drain. Finely mince the apricots with the raisins and sunflower seeds. Work the mixture well with your fingers.

Roll out the mixture between sheets of rice paper to a thickness of 6mm/¼in. Leave for 2 hours to set firm. Cut into 2.5cm/1in squares or small bars.

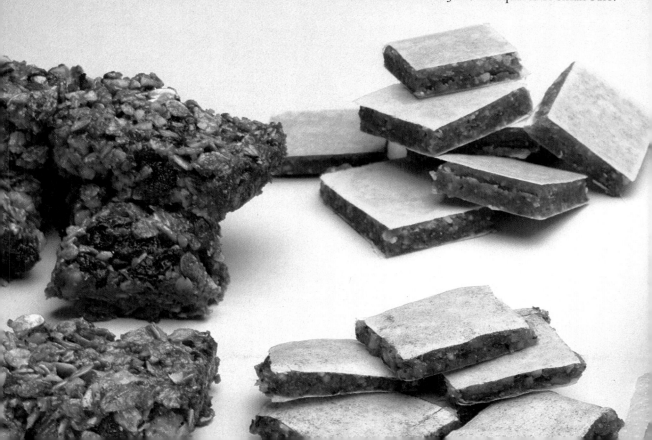

BAKING

Whenever you bake a cake, make pastry or biscuits or try your hand at homemade bread, wholewheat flour will give you delicious high-fibre results.

All types of cake can be made with wholewheat flour. Cakes do not rise quite so high as they do with white flour but they will have an excellent flavour so there is no need for elaborate icings or toppings.

When making wholewheat pastry you may find that you need a little more water than you do when using white flour and it may be a little more crumbly when you roll out the pastry. However, it should be just as light as white pastry, and pies made with wholewheat flour will be deep brown.

All biscuit and scone recipes can be made up with wholewheat flour without trouble. With scones, you will probably find that you will need less sugar than in your usual white flour recipe or even none at all, since using wholewheat flour gives them a delicious flavour of their own.

Wholewheat bread forms the basis of a well-balanced, high-fibre diet. Toast it for breakfast, make sandwich snacks and use the crumbs for stuffings and puddings.

The following recipes for bread all use fresh yeast. If only dried yeast is available, dissolve the honey or sugar in the warm water first, then sprinkle in the yeast. It takes about 20 minutes to begin to froth as opposed to 10 minutes for fresh yeast.

CORN OIL LEMON CAKE

175g/6 oz wholewheat flour
pinch of sea salt
1 tsp baking powder
grated rind of 1 lemon
150g/5 oz light Barbados sugar
125ml/4 fl oz corn oil
6 tbsp water
2 eggs, separated

FILLING
125g/4 oz curd cheese
3 tbsp sugar-free apricot jam

Heat the oven to 180°C/350°F/Gas 4. Put the flour into a bowl with the salt, baking powder, lemon rind and sugar. Mix together and make a well in the centre. Put in the oil, water and egg yolks. Beat everything together to make a fairly stiff mixture.

Stiffly whip the egg whites and fold into the rest. Put the mixture into 2 oiled 18cm/7in sponge tins and bake the cakes for 20 minutes so they are firm and have shrunk slightly from the sides of the tins. Turn the cakes onto wire racks to cool.

To make the filling, beat the cheese to a cream and beat in the jam, 1 tbsp at a time. Sandwich the two cakes together with the filling.

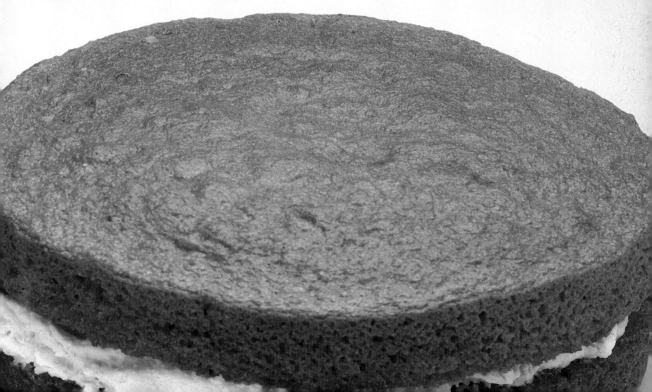

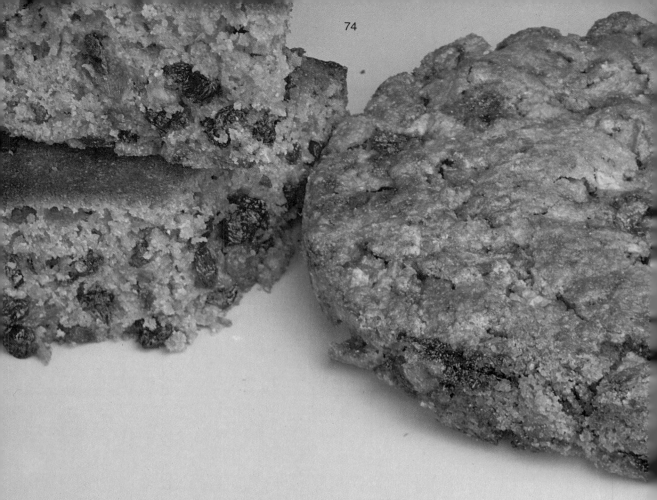

HONEY FRUIT CAKE

225g/8 oz butter
225g/8 oz honey
225g/8 oz wholewheat flour
1 tsp ground cinnamon
4 eggs, beaten
175g/6 oz sultanas
175g/6 oz raisins
25g/1 oz shelled walnuts, finely chopped
butter for greasing

Heat the oven to 180°C/350°F/Gas 4. Cream the
butter until soft and creamy. Stir in the honey and
beat until light and soft. Toss the flour with the
cinnamon and, alternately with the eggs, beat into
the butter and honey. Fold in the sultanas, raisins
and walnuts.

Put the mixture into a thickly buttered 20cm/8in
round cake tin and smooth the top. Bake the cake
for 50 minutes so it is golden brown on top and a
thin skewer stuck into the centre comes out clean.

Cool the cake for 10 minutes. Turn it onto a rack
to cool completely.

HOT APPLE CAKE

225g/8 oz wholewheat flour
½ nutmeg, grated
pinch of sea salt
1½ tsp baking powder
100g/4 oz lard plus extra for greasing
350g/12 oz Bramley apples
100g/4 oz molasses sugar
4 tbsp dry cider

Heat the oven to 180°C/350°F/Gas 4. Put the flour
into a bowl with the nutmeg, salt and baking
powder. Rub in the lard. Peel, core and finely chop
the apples and mix with the sugar. Mix the apples
and sugar into the flour with the cider.

Press the mixture into a greased 20-cm/8-in
diameter cake tin and bake the cake for 1 hour.

Turn out, cut into wedges and eat hot.

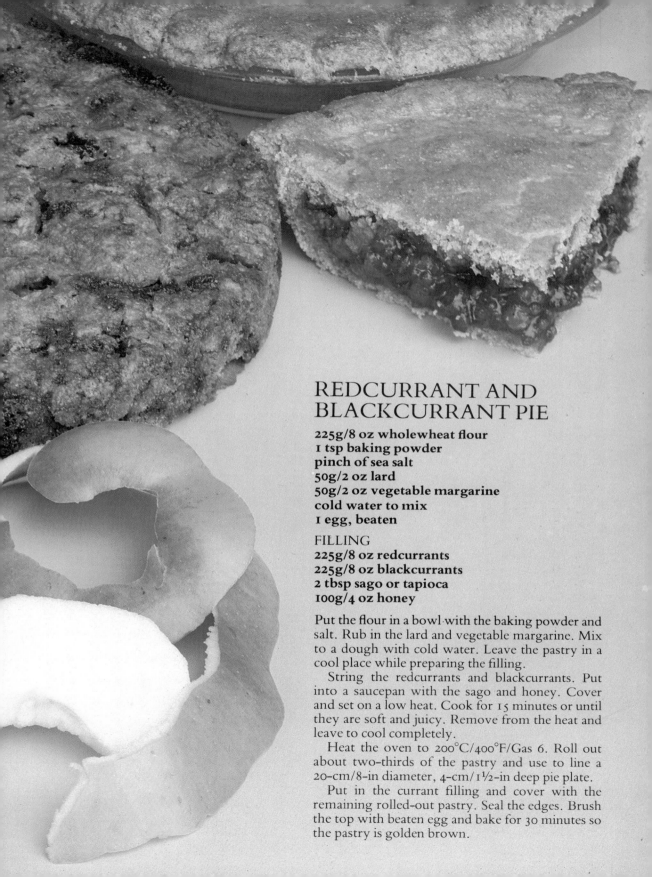

REDCURRANT AND BLACKCURRANT PIE

225g/8 oz wholewheat flour
1 tsp baking powder
pinch of sea salt
50g/2 oz lard
50g/2 oz vegetable margarine
cold water to mix
1 egg, beaten

FILLING
225g/8 oz redcurrants
225g/8 oz blackcurrants
2 tbsp sago or tapioca
100g/4 oz honey

Put the flour in a bowl with the baking powder and salt. Rub in the lard and vegetable margarine. Mix to a dough with cold water. Leave the pastry in a cool place while preparing the filling.

String the redcurrants and blackcurrants. Put into a saucepan with the sago and honey. Cover and set on a low heat. Cook for 15 minutes or until they are soft and juicy. Remove from the heat and leave to cool completely.

Heat the oven to 200°C/400°F/Gas 6. Roll out about two-thirds of the pastry and use to line a 20-cm/8-in diameter, 4-cm/1½-in deep pie plate.

Put in the currant filling and cover with the remaining rolled-out pastry. Seal the edges. Brush the top with beaten egg and bake for 30 minutes so the pastry is golden brown.

COCONUT BISCUITS

225g/8 oz wholewheat flour
75g/3 oz desiccated coconut
2 tsp baking powder
pinch of salt
1 tsp ground cinnamon
65g/2½ oz butter
75g/3 oz honey
1 egg, beaten

Heat the oven to 180°C/350°F/Gas 4. Put the flour into a bowl with the coconut, baking powder, salt and cinnamon. Make a well in the centre. Put the butter and honey into a saucepan and melt gently together. Pour into the flour. Add the egg and mix everything to a dough.

Roll out the dough to a thickness of 6mm/¼ in. Stamp into rounds with a 5cm/2in biscuit cutter. Put the biscuits on a floured baking sheet and bake for 20 minutes. Lift onto wire racks to cool.

WHOLEWHEAT BREAD

450g/1 lb wholewheat flour plus extra
for kneading
25g/1 oz fresh yeast
1 tsp honey or Barbados sugar
300ml/½ pint warm water
2 tsp sea salt
oil for greasing one 900g/2 lb loaf tin

Put the flour into a bowl. Cream the yeast with the honey or sugar and mix in half the water. Leave the yeast mixture in a warm place for about 10 minutes until it begins to froth. Dissolve the salt in the remaining water.

Make a well in the flour. Pour in the yeast mixture and mix in a little of the flour from the edges of the bowl. Pour in the salted water. Mix well. Turn the mixture onto a floured work surface and knead to a smooth dough. Return the dough to the bowl. Make a deep cross-cut in the top and cover the bowl with a clean tea cloth. Put into a warm place for 1 hour or until doubled in size.

Heat the oven to 200°C/400°F/Gas 6. Knead the dough again and lightly press into the prepared loaf tin. Cover with the cloth again and leave in a warm place until the dough has risen to the level of the sides of the tin. Bake the loaf for 50 minutes. Turn onto a wire rack to cool.

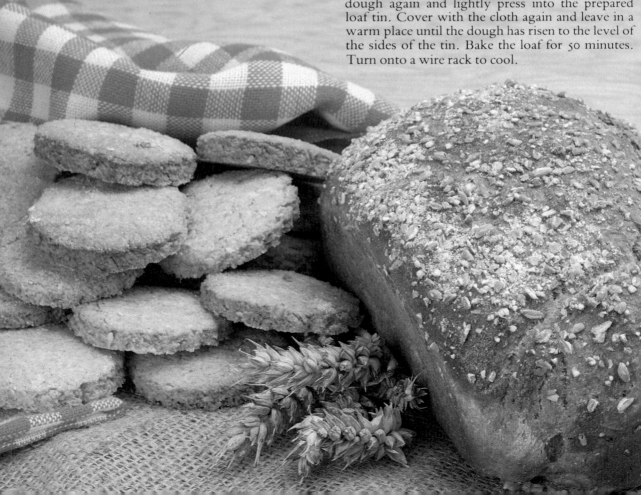

SAVOURY WALNUT SCONES

225g/8 oz wholewheat flour, plus extra for
    kneading
½ tsp bicarbonate of soda
1 tsp sea salt
40g/1½ oz butter
2 tbsp chopped parsley
1 tbsp chopped thyme
40g/1½ oz shelled walnuts, finely chopped
1 medium onion, finely chopped
150ml/¼ pint sour milk, buttermilk or
    natural yoghurt

Heat the oven to 200°C/400°F/Gas 6. Put the flour into a mixing bowl with the bicarbonate of soda and salt. Rub in 25g/1oz butter and mix in the herbs and walnuts.

Melt the remaining butter in a small frying pan on a low heat. Add the onion and cook until soft. Mix the onion into the flour. Make a well in the centre and pour in the sour milk, buttermilk or yoghurt. Mix everything to a dough. Turn it onto a floured work surface and knead lightly.

Roll the dough into a 2-cm/¾-in thick circle and cut into 8 triangles. Put onto a floured baking sheet and bake for 20 minutes.

Either eat hot or cool the scones on a wire rack.

SULTANA AND MALT LOAF

25g/1 oz fresh yeast
3 tbsp plus 1 tsp malt extract
150ml/¼ pint warm water
450g/1 lb wholewheat flour plus extra for
    kneading
2 tsp sea salt
50g/2 oz butter
175g/6 oz sultanas
150ml/¼ pint milk, warmed
butter or oil for greasing one 900g/2 lb loaf tin
1 egg, beaten
1 tbsp poppy seeds

Cream the yeast with 1 tsp malt extract and the water. Leave in a warm place for about 10 minutes until it begins to froth. Put the flour and salt into a bowl. Rub in the butter and toss in the sultanas. Make a well in the centre. Put in 3 tbsp malt extract and pour in the yeast mixture and the milk. Mix everything to a dough. Turn onto a floured work surface and knead. Return the dough to the bowl. Make a deep cross-cut in the top and cover the bowl with a clean tea cloth. Put into a warm place for 1 hour or until the dough has doubled in size.

Heat the oven to 200°C/400°F/Gas 6. Knead the dough again and put into the prepared loaf tin. Brush the top with beaten egg and scatter with poppy seeds. Slash down the centre with a sharp knife. Cover the loaf with the cloth and leave in a warm place for 15 minutes to prove. Bake the loaf for 50 minutes and turn onto a wire rack to cool.

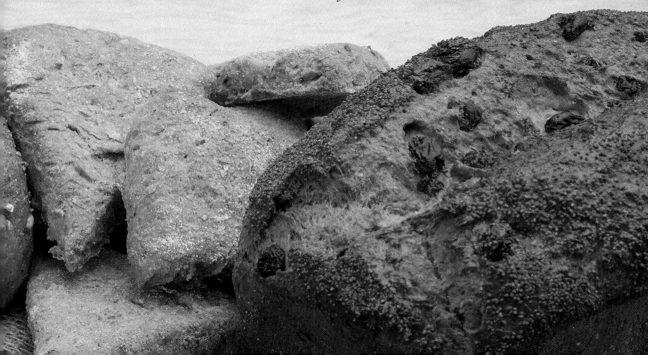

CHEESY ROLLS

2 tbsp skimmed milk powder
300ml/½ pint warm water
25g/1 oz fresh yeast
1 tsp honey
450g/1 lb wholewheat flour plus
   extra for kneading
2 tsp sea salt
150g/5 oz finely grated Cheddar cheese
1 egg, beaten
2 tbsp sesame seeds

Dissolve the milk powder in the warm water. Cream the yeast with the honey and stir in the milk. Leave the yeast in a warm place for about 10 minutes until it begins to froth. Put the flour and salt into a bowl. Rub in the cheese so it becomes well incorporated into the flour. Make a well in the centre and pour in the yeast mixture. Mix everything to a dough. Turn onto a floured work surface and knead until smooth. Return the dough to the bowl. Make a cross-cut in the top and cover the bowl with a clean tea cloth. Put into a warm place for 1 hour or until the dough has doubled in size.

Heat the oven to 200°C/400°F/Gas 6. Knead the dough again. Divide into 12 pieces and roll each one into a 25cm/10in rope. Roll each rope round in a spiral. Place the buns on a floured baking sheet. Brush with beaten egg and scatter with sesame seeds. Leave in a warm place for 10 minutes to prove. Bake for 20 minutes or until golden brown. Lift onto a wire rack to cool.

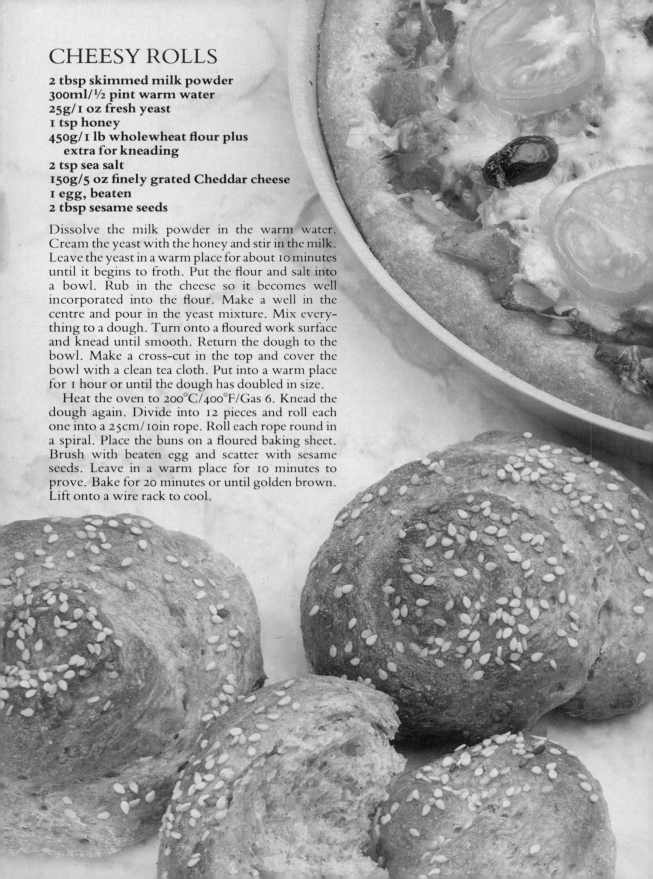

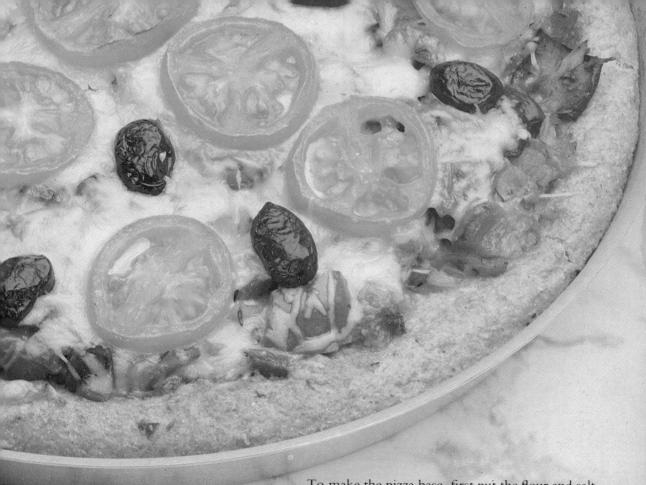

TUNA PIZZA

225g/8 oz wholewheat flour
½ tsp sea salt
20g/¾ oz fresh yeast or 15g/½ oz dried yeast
½ tsp Barbados sugar
6 tbsp warm water
1 egg, beaten
1 tbsp olive oil

FILLING
350g/12 oz aubergines
2 tbsp sea salt
one 200-g/7-oz tin tuna fish
2 green peppers
4 tbsp olive oil
1 large onion, finely chopped
1 garlic clove, finely chopped
2 tbsp tomato purée
1 tbsp chopped thyme
2 tbsp chopped parsley
75g/3 oz grated Edam cheese
225g/8 oz tomatoes, thinly sliced
6 black olives, halved and stoned

To make the pizza base, first put the flour and salt into a bowl. Cream the yeast with the sugar. Beat the water and egg together and mix into the yeast. Leave in a warm place for about 15–20 minutes until it begins to froth. Make a well in the centre of the flour. Mix in the yeast mixture and oil. Turn the dough back out onto a floured board and knead. Put the dough back into the bowl, cover with a cloth and put in a warm place to rise for 1 hour.

Dice the aubergines, put into a colander and sprinkle with salt. Leave for 20 minutes to drain. Rinse with cold water and dry with kitchen paper. Drain and flake the tuna fish. Core, seed and dice the peppers. Heat the oven to 200°C/400°F/Gas 6.

Heat the oil in a large frying pan on a low heat. Mix in the aubergines, peppers, onion and garlic and cook until the onion is soft. Mix in the tuna, tomato purée and herbs and remove the pan from the heat.

Knead the dough. Roll out to a 28cm/11in circle. Lay in the base of a 25cm/10in pizza tin and fold in the edges. Spread the tuna mixture over the base. Cover with the grated cheese and arrange the tomatoes and olives on top. Bake the pizza for 30 minutes.

INDEX